HYPERBARIC OXYGEN TREATMENT IN RESEARCH AND CLINICAL PRACTICE - MECHANISMS OF ACTION IN FOCUS

Edited by **Ines Drenjančević**

Hyperbaric Oxygen Treatment in Research and Clinical Practice - Mechanisms of Action in Focus
http://dx.doi.org/10.5772/intechopen.70322
Edited by Ines Drenjančević

Contributors

Edit Gara Dr, Ali Erdal Gunes, Gerardo Bosco, Alex Rizzato, Giuliano Vezzani, Vincenzo Zanon, Enrico Camporesi, Fethi Gul, Reyhan Arslantas, Omer Faruk Boran, Predrag Brkic, Sanja Pekovic, Sanja Dacic, Rada Jeremic, Marina Djelic, Danijela Krstic, Aleksandar Kibel, Ivana Jukić, Mihael Misir, Martina Mihalj, Zrinka Mihaljevic, Sanela Unfirer, Dijana Kibel, Ines Drenjančević

First published in London, United Kingdom, 2018 by IntechOpen
IntechOpen is the global imprint of INTECHOPEN LIMITED, registered in England and Wales, registration number: 11086078, The Shard, 25th floor, 32 London Bridge Street
London, SE19SG – United Kingdom
Printed in Croatia

British Library Cataloguing-in-Publication Data
A catalogue record for this book is available from the British Library

Additional hard copies can be obtained from orders@intechopen.com

Hyperbaric Oxygen Treatment in Research and Clinical Practice - Mechanisms of Action in Focus, Edited by Ines Drenjančević
p. cm.
Print ISBN 978-1-78923-598-2
Online ISBN 978-1-78923-599-9

For EU product safety concerns:
IN TECH d.o.o., Prolaz Marije Krucifikse Kozulić 3, 51000 Rijeka, Croatia,
info@intechopen.com or visit our website at intechopen.com.

Meet the editor

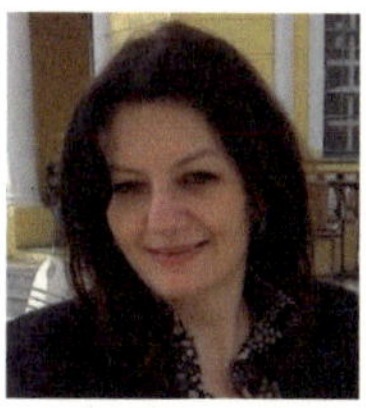

Ines Drenjančević, MD, PhD, is a tenure-track professor of Physiology and Immunology and the Chair of the Institute and Department of Physiology and Immunology, Faculty of Medicine Osijek, University Josip Juraj Strossmayer Osijek. She obtained her PhD degree in Physiology from the Medical College of Wisconsin, Milwaukee, Wisconsin, USA (2004) and MD degree (1993) and MS degree (1997) in Clinical Immunology and Allergology from the Faculty of Medicine University of Zagreb, Croatia. Her research has been funded at the national and international level. She is currently a PI of the Croatian Science Foundation project and a co-leader of the National Scientific Centre of Excellence for Personalized Health Care. Her interests include mechanisms of microvascular reactivity, effects of various diets (high salt intake, functional food, microelements) and hyperbaric oxygenation with the common denominator of oxygen sensing and metabolism of arachidonic acid.

Contents

Preface

The aim of this book, "Hyperbaric Oxygen Treatment in Research and Clinical Practice - Mechanisms of Action in Focus", is to present the current knowledge of the hyperbaric oxygen treatment in experimental research and clinical practice. There have been many controversies related to the HBO_2 protocols and indications, and our understanding on the mechanisms of HBO_2 action is still emerging. In April 2017, the Tenth European Consensus Conference on Hyperbaric Medicine was held, bringing consensus on accepted and non-accepted clinical indications and practices of hyperbaric oxygen treatment. Femoral neck necrosis is one of the indications for treatment with HBO_2 that received consensual Type 2 recommendation. This condition is described in the chapter "Therapeutic Mechanisms of Action for Hyperbaric Oxygen on Femoral Head Necrosis" by Gerardo Bosco et al. in this book. Sanja Pekovic et al. in the chapter "Hyperbaric Oxygen Therapy in Traumatic Brain Injury: Cellular and Molecular Mechanisms" describe HBO_2 as a potentially neuroprotective treatment and review a number of experimental and clinical studies on the mechanisms of traumatic brain injury. This indication receives Type 3 recommendation by the 10th EU Consensus Conference on Hyperbaric Medicine and is currently a field of intensive investigation both in basic medical sciences and in clinical trials.

Reduced microvascular perfusion is seen in many diseases, and hyperbaric oxygen treatment (HBO_2) has potentially beneficial effects on the microcirculatory environment. This topic is covered in the chapter "Microcirculation and Hyperbaric Oxygen Treatment" by Fethi Gul and co-authors. The chapter "Cell Culture Effects of Altered Oxygen Levels and Hyperbaric Treatment *In Vitro*" by Edit Gara deals with cell culture responses to HBO_2 and generally demonstrates the beneficial role of HBO_2 on proliferation and viability of most cell types. Furthermore, functional characteristics of the investigated cell types, e.g. angiogenesis by endothelial cell, are improved in response to HBO_2. Since oxygen is a highly reactive molecule and can induce upregulation of many various enzymatic systems in the cell, at the cellular, genetic and molecular level it can affect many cell functions. Particularly, vascular/endothelial function is affected by HBO_2. The chapter "Mechanisms of HBO-Induced Vascular Functional Changes in Diabetic Animal Models" by Ivana Jukic et al. describes the vascular functional changes affected by HBO_2 in animal model of diabetes mellitus.

And finally, as well as exhibiting beneficiary effects on the tissue perfusion, it is known that HBO_2 demonstrates high toxicity at higher pressures, due to increased oxidative stress and barotrauma. This is presented in the chapter "Toxic Effects of Hyperbaric Conditions" by Ali Erdal Gunes.

This book presents the reader with an overview of the current knowledge on the mechanisms of HBO_2 effects in various experimental models and clinical treatment protocols and open discussion on potentially new indications for HBO_2 and attempts to provide a better understanding of how and when HBO_2 should be used as an effective therapy without unwanted side effects.

Ines Drenjančević
Institute and Department of Physiology and Immunology
Faculty of Medicine Osijek
Josip Juraj Strossmayer University of Osijek, Croatia

Croatian National Scientific Center of Excellence for Personalized Health Care
Josip Juraj Strossmayer University of Osijek, Croatia

Chapter 1

Introductory Chapter: Hyperbaric Oxygen Treatment: Old Treatment with New Understanding

Ines Drenjančević

Additional information is available at the end of the chapter

http://dx.doi.org/10.5772/intechopen.79866

1. Introduction

Hyperbaric oxygen treatment (HBO_2) is a widely accepted adjuvant therapy in various health conditions that exhibit impaired tissue blood flow. The list of indications is widening as our knowledge and understanding on the mechanisms of HBO_2 action is getting larger. For example, in August 2013, the US Food and Drug Administration declared artery occlusion as one of the 13 specific indications for HBO therapy [1].

In April 2016, the Tenth European Consensus Conference on Hyperbaric Medicine was held, bringing consensus on accepted and non-accepted clinical indications and practice of hyperbaric oxygen treatment. Recommendations are listed in three levels of indications: from Type 1—strongly suggest that HBO_2 is to be accepted as primary treatment (example of accepted indications: carbon monoxide (CO) poisoning, mandibular osteonecrosis, gas embolism, anaerobic or mixed infections, decompression sickness, sudden deafness, etc.); Type 2—HBO_2 is suggested as it is supported by evidences (suggested indications: diabetic foot lesions, femoral head fracture, ischemic ulcers, etc.) and Type 3—where HBO_2 is optional, since it is not fully supported by evidences (e.g. brain injuries, radio-induced lesions, post-vascular procedure reperfusion syndrome, etc.). This consensus also provided negative recommendations, for example, where HBO_2 should not be used, such as autism spectrum disorders, placental insufficiency and cerebral palsy, to list some of them [2].

At high pressures, the delivery of the dissolved oxygen in plasma is enhanced, which contributes to better tissue oxygenation, cellular metabolism and, ultimately, healing. However, this is not the only potential mechanism for improved outcome of many diseases treated with HBO_2, since oxygen is highly reactive molecule and can induce upregulation of many various enzymatic systems in the cell, at cellular, genetic and molecular level. Particularly, vascular/endothelial function is affected by the HBO_2. Our understanding of these mechanisms of the HBO_2 effects is still emerging. There have been many controversies related to the HBO_2 protocols and indications. It is known that, as well as HBO_2 exhibit beneficiary effects on the tissue perfusion, it demonstrates high toxicity at higher pressures, due to increased oxidative stress and barotrauma. On the other hand, there is still a lack of the translation of the knowledge on the mechanisms of action of HBO_2 obtained from the experimental research to the clinical practice.

2. Effects of HBO_2 in brain injury

One interesting field of research of use of HBO_2 in treatment is brain injury, particularly traumatic brain injury and stroke in diabetes. In prospective, randomized controlled trial, in 79 diabetes patients suffering from acute intracerebral hemorrhagic stroke, both short-term and long-term neurological consequences were studied and compared in group on normobaric oxygen therapy and on HBO_2. At 1-month follow-up period, no distinct difference was observed between each group. However, after 6 months of follow-up, HBO_2 group exhibited better neurological consequences compared to control group (Barthel Index: 85.1 versus 65.6%, P = 0.080; mRS: 89.4 versus 68.8%, P = 0.045; Glasgow outcome scale: 83.0 versus 62.5%, P = 0.073; National Institute of Stroke Scale (NIHSS): 80.9 versus 56.2%, P = 0.035), supporting the hypothesis that HBO_2 is safe and effective therapy for the long-term neurological outcomes in diabetic patients with hemorrhagic stroke [3].

In traumatic brain injury (TBI) clinical study, 28 patients with persistent cognitive impairment caused by mild-to-moderate TBI were included and examined for the stem cell mobilization and recruitment to repair damaged neuronal tissue. HBO_2 treatment correlated with stem cell mobilization as well as increased cognitive performance. The limitation of the study was that peripheral blood sample was tested [4]. Similarly, 50 randomized subjects with TBI were examined for cognition and post-traumatic stress disorder symptoms. They completed a total of 30 HBO_2 exposures compared to sham-treated group. The symptoms improved in both groups and there were no statistically significant differences between groups. However, there was some improvement in the treatment group versus the control after subgroup analyses based on concussion history and individual test components [5]. In randomized controlled clinical trial, normobaric oxygen therapy was also employed in the treatment of 52 patients with either ischemic or hemorrhagic stroke in the first 12 h of accident. Normobaric oxygenation could improve long-time outcome of the patients based on the modified Rankin Scale neurology disability scoring system, but not on the Barthel results, 6 months after the discharge from hospital [6]. The retrospective observational trial demonstrated significant improvement in patients with acute neurological deficits due to ischemic stroke following cardiac surgery treated with HBO_2. However, the last study lacks control, which weakens the level of evidence of conclusions [7].

Contrary to this beneficiary results, recent Cochrane database systemic review included 11 randomized clinical trials (RCTs) involving 705 participants to examine the effect of HBO_2

on clinical outcomes of ischemic stroke. Fatality rate at 6 months was not significantly different in those receiving HBO_2 compared with the control group. However, HBO_2 significantly improved 4 of 14 scale measures of disability and functional performance, for example, the mean Orgogozo Scale score was higher (MD 27.9 points, 95% CI 4.0–51.8, P value 0.02) and Trouillas Disability Scale score was lower with HBO_2 (mean difference (MD) 2.2 point reduction with HBOT, 95% CI 0.15–4.3, P value 0.04). The limiting factor of this meta-analysis was variable quality of the methodology of the evaluated trials; thus, it is not conclusive on clear clinical benefit as well as on exclusion of it [8].

Analyses of several trials, such as the Department of Defense/Veterans Administration (DoD/VA) sponsored trials, previous published reports on the use of HBO_2 therapy on stroke and moderate chronic traumatic brain injury (mTBI) and preliminary reports from the HOPPS Army trial, suggest the approval of HBO_2 for neurological indications, especially for mTBI and post-concussion syndrome (PCS), as a safe and viable treatment for recovery in the post-acute phase [9]. In the context of the preparation of impending National Institute of Neurologic Disorders and Stroke-funded, multi-center, randomized, adaptive Phase II clinical trial—the Hyperbaric Oxygen Brain Injury Treatment (HOBIT) trial, 30 studies (8 clinical and 22 pre-clinical) that administered HBO_2 within 30 days of a TBI were analyzed. The pre-clinical studies consistently reported positive treatment effects across a variety of outcome measures with almost no safety concerns. Of the eight clinical studies reviewed, four were based on the senior author's (GR) investigation of HBO_2 as a treatment for acute severe TBI [10].

The mechanisms by which HBO_2 induces brain neuroplasticity can be demonstrated by highly sensitive MRI techniques of dynamic susceptibility contrast-enhanced (DSC) and diffusion tensor imaging (DTI). Fifteen patients afflicted with prolonged post-concussion syndrome were treated with 60 daily HBO_2 sessions. The cerebral blood flow and volume significantly increased after HBO_2. There was significant improvement in the memory, information processing speed, executive functions and global cognitive scores (evaluated by NeuroTrax) after HBO_2. Fractional anisotropy values were significantly increased and mean diffusivity was significantly decreased in both white and gray matter structures after HBO_2 [11].

Hyperbaric oxygen in combination with thrombolysis shows neuroprotection in acute ischemic stroke in rats by reducing infarct volume and improving functional outcome in the early post-stroke period [12]. HBO_2 can induce cerebral angiogenesis and improve both white and gray microstructures indicating regeneration of nerve fibers which correlates with the neurocognitive improvements [11]. Potential metabolic effects in the mechanisms of HBO_2-induced improved neurostructural and neurofunctional outcomes were also examined in diabetic female rats. Particular emphasis was given to the role of cyp450 enzymes' metabolites of arachidonic acid. Cortical infarct size and total infarct size were equally and significantly reduced in HBO_2- and HET0016 (inhibitor of 20-HETE production)-treated diabetic female rats. Cyp2J3 mRNA was significantly increased in all study groups, and Cyp2C11 mRNA was significantly increased in the group receiving HET0016 treatment followed by HBO_2 exposure and in the multiple HBO_2 group compared to the control group. Endothelial nitric oxide synthase (eNOS) enzyme's expression was significantly increased after HBO_2 treatments, and expression of epoxide hydrolase 2 was increased in all groups compared to the control group. All together, these results suggested that cytochrome P450 metabolites and the NO pathway are involved in the observed therapeutic effects of HBO_2 and HET0016 in diabetic female Sprague-Dawley rats. Furthermore, HBO_2 and HET0016 are very effective treatments of stroke [13]. Similarly, HBO_2 treatment on rats with experimental traumatic spinal cord injury was performed 1, 6 and 24 h after brain trauma. HBO_2 improved the results of the inclined plane level tests and motor strength test. Early HBO_2 treatment resulted in higher recovery rates, particularly when treatment started in the first hour. In traumatized rats, nitrite levels in spinal cord increased compared to control group; however, they diminished after HBO_2 treatments. As earlier the HBO_2 treatment was conducted, the greater decrease in nitrite levels was observed [14].

The safety of more advanced attempts to deliver increased oxygen levels to hypoxic or ischemic tissues, such as with hyperbaric oxygen therapy, is also being questioned [15]. There are substantial number of evidence that HBO_2 significantly improves physiologic measures without causing cerebral or pulmonary toxicity and can potentially improve clinical outcome [10]. In contrast to chronic, intermittent HBO_2 treatments which do not increase oxidative stress and restore the mechanisms of vascular relaxation in diabetic rats [16, 17], acute HBO_2 can increase oxidative stress and transiently impair the endothelium-dependent vasorelaxation, even in healthy rats [18]. In study on isolated aortic rings in healthy male Sprague-Dawley rats, acetylcholine-induced relaxation and hypoxia-induced relaxation which were impaired after acute HBO_2 due to increased serum oxidative stress and superoxide production were restored by superoxide scavenger TEMPOL. The mRNA expression of iNOS was decreased in the acute HBO_2 and 24 h after HBO_2 while gene expression of superoxide dismutase SOD1 and SOD3 and NADPH oxidase was increased in the intermittent HBO_2 group. The expression and activity of catalase and glutathione peroxidase were increased in the intermittent HBO_2 group as well. Vasorelaxation was restored and oxidative stress was normalized 24 h after the treatment [18].

In attempt to evaluate possibility to use HBO_2 in other neurological diseases, such as Alzheimer's disease (AD), the studies were performed in the triple transgenic model of AD in old mice. HBO_2 reduced hypoxia, amyloid burden and tau phosphorylation in 3xTg mice and ameliorated their behavioral deficits. HBO_2 attenuated neuroinflammatory processes by reducing astrogliosis, microgliosis and the secretion of proinflammatory cytokines (IL-1β and TNFα) and increasing expression of scavenger receptor A, arginase1 and anti-inflammatory cytokines (IL-4 and IL-10) [19]. The beneficial effect of HBO_2 for neurological outcome after stroke has been illustrated in many studies, and meanwhile, many underlying mechanisms associated with neuroprotection have been demonstrated, such as cerebral oxygenation promotion and metabolic improvement, decreased oxidative stress and apoptosis, blood-brain barrier protection, anti-inflammation and decrease in cerebral edema, intracranial pressure modulation and increased vascular and neural regeneration [20]. However, as noted previously, studies performed in human stroke patients lack controls. Thus, data are not sufficiently evidence-based, although promising. In human stroke, there is an urgent need for the randomized double-blind controlled clinical trials to have undoubted evidence on the HBO_2 effects in stroke. In the future, this type of studies will lead to uniform criteria on the dose, number of sessions and oxygenation levels in different types of stroke.

3. Potential HBO_2 use in inflammatory bowel diseases

Another interesting and controversial field of potential HBO_2 application is inflammatory bowel diseases and radiation-induced chronic gastrointestinal symptoms. Again, some studies presented beneficiary effects of HBO_2 in the model of ulcerative colitis, by stimulating colonic stem cells to promote healing. However, this study lack control group [21]. On the other hand, well-controlled study in mice model of DSS-induced colitis demonstrated that HBO_2 significantly reduces colitis severity. Gene expression and activity of antioxidative enzymes were changed by the HBO_2, as well as the inflammatory microenvironment in the gut mucosa. This was manifested by the clinical features of colitis (e.g. bleeding, frequency of stool) and by histological assessment of the gut tissue and reversal of IL-1β, IL-2 and IL-6 gene expression. Also, the immune cell expansion and mobilization were impaired. HIF-1α mRNA level strongly correlated to GPx1, SOD1 and IL-6 mRNA expression, suggesting that HIF-1α is involved in the transcriptional regulation of these genes during colonic inflammation and HBO_2 [22]. On the other hand, a prospective randomized study failed to demonstrate that HBO_2 can improve the effects of standardized treatment in a severe attack of ulcerative colitis [23]. Additionally, no evidence that patients with radiation-induced chronic gastrointestinal symptoms, including those patients with rectal bleeding, benefit from hyperbaric oxygen therapy in HOT2 study (a double-blind, sham-controlled, phase 3 randomized study of patients (≥18 years) with chronic gastrointestinal symptoms for 12 months or more after radiotherapy) [24]. Obviously, there is a discrepancy of the data from experimental study and clinical observational studies, which need to be resolved by well-controlled randomized clinical trials and well-settled experimental studies.

4. Conclusion

HBO_2 is an established therapeutic approach in many acute, life-threatening conditions and also has been submitted to scrutinizing evaluation for new indications. Not only there is a wide field of potential application of HBO_2 in experimental research and clinical therapy, but also there is a need for improved understanding of the mechanisms of action of HBO_2. Mechanisms of HBO_2-induced beneficiary effects are under intense investigation and their understanding promise HBO_2 with low unwanted side effects when utilized in well-designed controlled fashion.

Author details

Ines Drenjančević[1,2*]

*Address all correspondence to: ines.drenjancevic@mefos.hr

1 Institute and Department of Physiology and Immunology, Faculty of Medicine Osijek, Josip Juraj Strossmayer University of Osijek, Osijek, Croatia

2 Croatian National Scientific Center of Excellence for Personalized Health Care, Josip Juraj Strossmayer University of Osijek, Osijek, Croatia

References

[1] Ding Z, Tong WC, Lu XX, Peng HP. Hyperbaric oxygen therapy in acute ischemic stroke: A review. Interventional Neurology. 2014;**2**(4):201-211. DOI: 10.1159/000362677

[2] Mathieu D, Marroni A, Kot J. Tenth European consensus conference on hyperbaric medicine: Recommendations for accepted and non-accepted clinical indications and practice of hyperbaric oxygen treatment. Diving and Hyperbaric Medicine. 2017;**47**(1):24-32. DOI: 10.28920/dhm47.1.24-32

[3] Xu Q, Fan SB, Wan YL, Liu XL, Wang L. The potential long-term neurological improvement of early hyperbaric oxygen therapy on hemorrhagic stroke in the diabetics. Diabetes Research and Clinical Practice. 2018;**138**:75-80. DOI: 10.1016/j.diabres.2018.01.017

[4] Shandley S, Wolf EG, Schubert-Kappan CM, Baugh LM, Richards MF, Prye J, Arizpe HM, Kalns J. Increased circulating stem cells and better cognitive performance in traumatic brain injury subjects following hyperbaric oxygen therapy. Undersea and Hyperbaric Medicine. 2017;**44**(3):257-269

[5] Wolf EG, Baugh LM, Kabban CM, Richards MF, Prye J. Cognitive function in a traumatic brain injury hyperbaric oxygen randomized trial. Undersea and Hyperbaric Medicine. 2015;**42**(4):313-332

[6] Mazdeh M, Taher A, Torabian S, Seifirad S. Effects of normobaric hyperoxia in severe acute stroke: A randomized controlled clinical trial study. Acta Medica Iranica. 2015;**53**(11):676-680

[7] Weixler VH, Yates AE, Puchinger M, Zirngast B, Pondorfer P, Ratzenhofer-Komenda B, Amegah-Sakotnik A, Smolle-Juettner FM, Dapunt O. Hyperbaric oxygen in patients with ischemic stroke following cardiac surgery: A retrospective observational trial. Undersea and Hyperbaric Medicine. 2017;**44**(5):377-385

[8] Bennett MH, Weibel S, Wasiak J, Schnabel A, French C, Kranke P. Hyperbaric oxygen therapy for acute ischaemic stroke. Cochrane Database of Systematic Reviews. Nov 12, 2014;**11**:CD004954. DOI: 10.1002/14651858.CD004954.pub3

[9] Figueroa XA, Wright JK. Clinical results in brain injury trials using HBO_2 therapy: Another perspective. Undersea and Hyperbaric Medicine. Jul–Aug 2015;**42**(4):333-351

[10] Daly S, Thorpe M, Rockswold S, Hubbard M, et al. Hyperbaric oxygen therapy in the treatment of acute severe traumatic brain injury: A systematic review. Journal of Neurotrauma. Feb 15, 2018;**35**(4):623-629. DOI: 10.1089/neu.2017.5225

[11] Tal S, Hadanny A, Sasson E, Suzin G, Efrati S. Hyperbaric oxygen therapy can induce angiogenesis and regeneration of nerve fibers in traumatic brain injury patients. Frontiers in Human Neuroscience. Oct 19, 2017;**11**:508. DOI: 10.3389/fnhum.2017.00508

[12] Küppers-Tiedt L, Manaenko A, Michalski D, Guenther A, Hobohm C, Wagner A, Zhang JH, Schneider D. Combined systemic thrombolysis with alteplase and early hyperbaric oxygen therapy in experimental embolic stroke in rats: Relationship to functional outcome and reduction of structural damage. Acta Neurochirurgica. Supplement. 2011;**111**:167-172. DOI: 10.1007/978-3-7091-0693-8_28

[13] Mišir M, Renić M, Novak S, Mihalj M, Ćosić A, Vesel M, Drenjančević I. Hyperbaric oxygenation and 20-hydroxyeicosatetreanoic acid inhibition reduce stroke volume in female diabetic Sprague-Dawley rats. Experimental Physiology. 2017;**102**(12):1596-1606. DOI: 10.1113/EP086402

[14] Yaman O, Yaman B, Aydın F, Var A, Temiz C. Hyperbaric oxygen treatment in the experimental spinal cord injury model. The Spine Journal. 2014;**14**(9):2184-2194. DOI: 10.1016/j.spinee.2014.02.013

[15] Sjöberg F1, Singer M. The medical use of oxygen: A time for critical reappraisal. Journal of Internal Medicine. 2013;**274**(6):505-528. DOI: 10.1111/joim.12139

[16] Unfirer S, Mihalj M, Novak S, Kibel A, Cavka A, Mihaljevic Z, Gros M, Brizic I, Budimir D, Cosic A, Boban M, Drenjancevic I. Hyperbaric oxygenation affects the mechanisms of acetylcholine-induced relaxation in diabetic rats. Undersea and Hyperbaric Medicine. 2016;**43**(7):787-803

[17] Kibel A, Novak S, Cosic A, Mihaljevic Z, Falck JR, Drenjancevic I. Hyperbaric oxygenation modulates vascular reactivity to angiotensin-(1-7) in diabetic rats: Potential role of epoxyeicosatrienoic acids. Diabetes and Vascular Disease Research. 2015;**12**(1):33-45. DOI: 10.1177/1479164114553424

[18] Mihaljević Z, Matić A, Stupin A, Rašić L, Jukić I, Drenjančević I. Acute hyperbaric oxygenation, contrary to intermittent hyperbaric oxygenation, adversely affects Vasorelaxation in healthy Sprague-Dawley rats due to increased oxidative stress. Oxidative Medicine and Cellular Longevity. 2018;**29**(2018):7406027. DOI: 10.1155/2018/7406027

[19] Shapira R, Solomon B, Efrati S, Frenkel D, Ashery U. Hyperbaric oxygen therapy ameliorates pathophysiology of 3xTg-AD mouse model by attenuating neuroinflammation. Neurobiology of Aging. 2018;**62**:105-119. DOI: 10.1016/j.neurobiolaging.2017.10.007

[20] Zhai WW, Sun L, Yu ZQ, Chen G. Hyperbaric oxygen therapy in experimental and clinical stroke. Medical Gas Research. Jul 11, 2016;**6**(2):111-118

[21] Bekheit M, Baddour N, Katri K, Taher Y, El Tobgy K, Mousa E. Hyperbaric oxygen therapy stimulates colonic stem cells and induces mucosal healing in patients with refractory ulcerative colitis: A prospective case series. BMJ Open Gastroenterology. 2016;**3**(1):e000082. DOI: 10.1136/bmjgast-2016-000082

[22] Novak S, Drenjancevic I, Vukovic R, Kellermayer Z, Cosic A, Tolusic Levak M, Balogh P, Culo F, Mihalj M. Anti-inflammatory effects of hyperbaric oxygenation during DSS-induced colitis in BALB/c mice include changes in gene expression of HIF-1α, proinflammatory cytokines, and antioxidative enzymes. Mediators of Inflammation. 2016; **2016**:7141430

[23] Pagoldh M, Hultgren E, Arnell P, Eriksson A. Hyperbaric oxygen therapy does not improve the effects of standardized treatment in a severe attack of ulcerative colitis: A prospective randomized study. Scandinavian Journal of Gastroenterology. 2013;**48**(9): 1033-1040. DOI: 10.3109/00365521.2013.819443

[24] Glover M, Smerdon GR, Andreyev HJ, Benton BE, Bothma P, Firth O, Gothard L, Harrison J, Ignatescu M, Laden G, Martin S, Maynard L, McCann D, Penny CEL, Phillips S, Sharp G, Yarnold J. Hyperbaric oxygen for patients with chronic bowel dysfunction after pelvic radiotherapy (HOT2): A randomised, double-blind, sham-controlled phase 3 trial. The Lancet Oncology. 2016;**17**(2):224-233. DOI: 10.1016/S1470-2045(15)00461-1

Chapter 2

Therapeutic Mechanisms of Action for Hyperbaric Oxygen on Femoral Head Necrosis

Gerardo Bosco, Alex Rizzato, Giuliano Vezzani,
Vincenzo Zanon and Enrico Camporesi

Additional information is available at the end of the chapter

http://dx.doi.org/10.5772/intechopen.75026

Abstract

Femoral head necrosis (FHN) is a disease process resulting from inadequate blood perfusion of subchondral bone. While the etiology of this disease is still not fully understood, there are multiple traumatic and atraumatic factors that are associated with the disease. Pathophysiology of the disease is characterized by the death of bone marrow and osteocytes. If left untreated, the disease may progress to joint collapse. While initial stages of the disease are asymptomatic, painful limitation of active and passive motion of the hip is eventually present. The current body of literature cannot identify an optimal treatment protocol for FHN. Postcollapse cases require surgical intervention, core decompression, or total hip arthroplasty. However, current strides in conservative management are being made. One of the possible conservative modalities that may effectively delay hip arthroplasty or even prevent the need for a surgical approach is hyperbaric oxygen (HBO_2) therapy. HBO_2 increases extracellular oxygen concentration and reduces cellular ischemia and edema by inducing vasoconstriction. Studies have reported radiographic improvement, reduction in pain, and increases in range of motion for early stages of the disease. Hyperbaric oxygen therapy has also been shown to stimulate angiogenesis and enhance osteoclast and osteoblast function for remodeling and repair.

Keywords: hyperbaric oxygen, femoral head necrosis, mechanisms of action, inflammation, cytokines

1. Introduction

Femoral head necrosis (FHN), also named avascular necrosis or osteonecrosis of the femoral head, is a common multifactorial disorder that affects patients of any age and can result in substantial clinical morbidity [1]. Osteonecrosis is characterized by the lack of or inadequate blood flow to the bony tissue that leads to death of the osteocytes and the bone marrow [2].

As reported by Parsons and colleagues, it is most common in the second to fifth decades of life, and the typical patient is a male, in his mid-30s [3]. Epidemiology reveals between 10,000 and 20,000 new cases of FHN diagnosed each year in the United States [4]. In the western countries, the prevalence of the disease is at a mean age of 39 years, and the 10% of hip replacements performed is due to FHN [5]. Femoral head collapse, hip joint degenerative lesions, and subsequent long-term disability represent possible adverse consequences of the untreated or nondiagnosed FHN [6]. In particular, it is estimated that more than 70% of femoral heads with osteonecrosis will proceed to collapse, requiring prosthetic joint replacement within 3–4 years of diagnosis [7]. About that, it is responsible for 5–18% of all hip replacements performed [4]. Moreover, similar pathophysiology can occur in other articular districts (i.e., the femoral condyle, the wrist, the head of the humerus, and the distal talus) caused by comparable avascular syndromes. Multifocal osteonecrosis is defined as a disease involving three or more separate anatomic sites concurrently or consecutively [8].

Radiographic diagnosis is now possible at a former stage; thus, orthopedic physicians can identify the disorder earlier [9].

Hyperbaric oxygen (HBO) therapy is one of the proposed treatments. Indeed, tissue oxygenation promotes angiogenesis inducing edema reduction [1]. Moreover, by reducing intraosseous pressure, venous drainage is restored and the microcirculation is improved [10]. With restriction to the stage considered, Camporesi et al. showed that HBO should be considered the primary treatment modality in any patients and especially in young patients where the goal is to delay total hip arthroplasty as long as possible [5]. Therefore, the European Community accepted femoral head necrosis as an indication for hyperbaric oxygen therapy (HBOT) during the Consensus Conference in Lille, France [11].

Originally, the relation between femoral head necrosis and HBOT was deeply analyzed on a specific chapter published on Hyperbaric Medicine Practice [12]. It reported precise charts of patient results and a detailed review of the literature until 1997, as well as the different pathological outcomes and rationale for treatment [13]. Recently, an extended report on this topic has been proposed by Bosco and colleagues [1, 14]. They precisely updated the scientific literature until 2016 and summarized, for the paper's eligibility for the study, the number of patients, aim, inclusion/exclusion criteria, and obtained outcomes. Even though management, care, and therapeutic options are clearly stated for the pathology, available results differ from each other according to the stratification criteria and the particular stage of the disorder [15]. The present chapter aims to review more recent evidence from the scientific literature, outlining the physiology and the present status of pathology and therapy for femoral head necrosis. In particular, we focused on therapeutic mechanisms of action for hyperbaric oxygen (HBO_2) on femoral head necrosis.

2. Etiology

In studying FHN, the absence of a bipedal mammalian model limits our knowledge among risk factors and pathogenesis of the disease. Additionally, completing longitudinal studies is difficult for researchers and clinicians. However, scientific community agrees that ischemia plays a main role in the pathogenesis. As aforementioned, FHN is a multifactorial disease in which both genetic and daily-living factors lead to the pathology. When evaluating patients with osteonecrosis, physicians should first differentiate between primary ("idiopathic") osteonecrosis and secondary osteonecrosis [16]. Although the etiology of secondary osteonecrosis has not been clearly delineated, risk factors include both traumatic and nontraumatic conditions (i.e., corticosteroid use, alcohol consumption, smoking, coagulation abnormalities, etc.) [17].

Traumatic events may lead to bone fracture or at worst to femoral head displacement; since the trauma occurs, it directly results in disruption of the femoral head blood supply [18]. Malizos et al. distinguished different pathogeneses in patients with subcapital fracture and patients with hip dislocation. In the first case, the 10–20% of the vascularization of femoral head is preserved from ligamentum teres. Conversely, as the hip dislocation occurs, blood supply is interrupted, and perfusion depends on the integrity of retinacular vessels [2].

Otherwise, nontraumatic osteonecrosis is frequently associated with pathologies where corticosteroid treatment is required (i.e., systemic lupus erythematosus, organ transplant, lymphoma, etc.). A report described the case of a female patient who was just under 18 years old when she underwent surgery due to bilateral osteonecrosis of the femoral condyles that developed in the course of treatment of a hematological malignancy [19]. Even though, scientific literature does not know the exact dose of steroids necessary to induce osteonecrosis, the higher the dose the greater the risk. Indeed, daily mean or peak dose taken seems to be more implicated than cumulative or duration of therapy [3]. Furthermore, an addiction to alcohol and long drinking period were reported as risk factors for FHN. In comparing gender difference, studies indicated for males a greater frequency of alcohol-induced FHN with respect to females [20, 21]. Indeed, Shimizu et al. showed a bigger susceptibility of males in developing FHN in response to alcohol consumption. Specifically, females did not develop osteonecrosis for alcohol consumption for both short-time and long-time periods. However, further investigations are needed among sex-related factors responsible for this evidence [20].

Further risk factors of FHN can be identified in bone marrow transplantation, as well as metastatic malignancies, and pregnancy. Additionally, it may be associated with pathologies as hyperuricemia, pancreatitis, and leukemia or lymphoma [9, 14].

3. Pathophysiology

FHN physiopathology is characterized from a complex series of events that couple a usual pathway of cellular death and osteogenic processes [14]. Pathogenic course begins with two associated mechanisms: edema of interstitial marrow and necrosis of hematopoietic cells and adipocytes. Histological signs appear nearly 24–72 h following anoxia, even though osteocyte necrosis is evident after approximately 2–3 h of oxygen deprivation [22, 23]. These stimuli induce bone remodeling processes. Originally, inflammatory signs (i.e., reactive hyperemia and capillary revascularization) surround the necrotic area. Thus, this mechanism initiates bone repairing in which new bone hardly tries to remove and substitute dead tissues [9].

However, bone remodeling proceeds inefficiently because of dead trabeculae, where new living bone is placed. Moreover, osteolysis exceeds osteogenesis, and this results in loss of structural integrity of trabeculae, with subsequent subchondral fracture and joint incongruity [24].

Altered subchondral vascularity is the basic pathophysiological hallmark for FHN [9]. Kiaer and colleagues indicated that a blood supply drop of 60% will result in an intraosseous pO_2 decrease, from 75 mmHg to 50 mmHg [25]. Consequently, it will cause evident ischemia.

Different pathogenic mechanisms can result in FHN. Cytotoxicity due to exposure to radiation, chemotherapy, or thermal injury causes direct death of marrow cells and osteocytes, though this was not shown in vivo yet [18]. Additionally, three main pathogenic mechanisms can lead to ischemic conditions and subsequent femoral head necrosis:

1. Vascular interruption by fractures or dislocation (i.e., traumatic osteonecrosis). Femoral neck fractures or hip displacement usually result in extra-osseous arterial involvement. Specifically, when fracture occurs inside the joint capsule, vessels that oxygenate the subchondral bone suffer a direct trauma. A relatively high incidence of FHN in patients with these fractures has been reported.

2. Intravascular coagulation and microcirculatory thrombosis. Different pathways can lead to the same vascular obstructions that mean sickle cell aggregations, clots, or lipid thrombi [6]. Thrombotic emboli can occur both in arteriosus and venous areas in samples of osteonecrotic tissue; in some animal models, they have been associated with osteocyte necrosis [3]. The prevalence of sickle cell anemia-induced osteonecrosis stands between 37 and 50%. The weak arterial network in the hip joint eases vascular occlusion by sickled cells [16]. In these patients, low oxygen tension environments are hypothesized to trigger hemoglobin precipitation which leads to erythrocyte sickling [6]. Moreover, the complication rate for patients with sickle cell disease undergoing orthopedic procedures is significantly higher than that for patients without sickle disease. Consequently, early and alternative interventions are critical to successfully delay total hip arthroplasty.

   Also, coagulation disorders are implicated in FHN. For example, genetic defects resulting in hypofibrinolysis or thrombophilia may lead to increased thrombi formation and blood flow obstruction in the bony tissues. Nevertheless, using a case-control methodology, elevated coagulation factor levels have been reported in patients with osteonecrosis showing the absence of known genetic defects [14]. Jarman et al. showed that coagulation abnormality-derived osteonecrosis is worsened by testosterone therapy, and its development may be slowed or stopped by discontinuation of therapy and, thereafter, anticoagulation [26]. Indeed, Guo and colleagues suggested the use of anticoagulant therapy for primary FHN. However, anticoagulants cannot play a protective role on secondary FHN [27]. Coagulation pathologies recognized before femoral head necrosis simplify therapeutic approach, preserving joints.

3. Intraosseous extravascular compression from lipocyte hypertrophy or Gaucher cells. It can also result from hemorrhage, infection, high bone marrow pressure, marrow infiltration, and bone marrow edema [18]. Physiologically, since the pressure increases within

the intraosseous extravascular region, microcirculation in vessels crossing the tissue decreases. Nevertheless, it is not a regular event. Many times, steroid consumption influences lipid metabolism leading to fat production in bone stem cells and drug-induced osteoporosis and osteonecrosis [3, 28]. This process will soon result in fat cell hypertrophy. Subsequently, intraosseous pressure will rise and ischemic condition will occur [29]. Though osteonecrosis is mostly associated with hypercholesterolemia and/or hypertriglyceridemia, the osteonecrosis-related lipid abnormalities have been well documented with the Gaucher disease (GD) [16]. Gaucher disease (GD) is a lysosomal storage disorder, caused by an impaired function of β-glucocerebrosidase, which results in accumulation of glucocerebroside in cells, and altered membrane ordering [30]. However, microcirculatory blood flow blockage is not necessarily the starting pathological event. Lysosomal contents released from Gaucher cells may damage vessel membrane, with localized osteonecrosis that may extend to bordering areas [31]. Skeletal involvement is typical in mature patients suffering from type 1 Gaucher disease, with a radiological evidence described in 93% of cases. Among these, the 30% presents osteonecrosis [31].

4. The fourth physiopathological mechanism is under investigation: extra-osseous venous obstruction. Although impairment of the extra-osseous veins happens, there is still an uncertainty whether it is a cause or effect. Additionally, it possibly has limited clinical meaning [6]. Recently, Shah et al. reviewed literature on this topic, and they investigated increased intraosseous pressure as a pathogenic process in FHN. In particular, bloodstream interruption or stasis in the venous side has been associated with increased pressure in osteonecrotic samples [6].

Since the seventies, scholars studied dysbaric osteonecrosis and explained radiographic features of this pathology [32]. It is an avascular bone necrosis induced by exposure to hyperbaric environments, typical for diverse and compressed air workers [33]. A literature review on dysbaric osteonecrosis evidenced that incomplete decompression procedures lead to blood supply decrease and subsequent osteonecrosis; this is due to the entry of nitrogen bubbles in the fatty marrow-containing shafts of long bones [34]. Studies clearly stated the approach to be used, outlining diving decompression schedules [33].

4. Rationale for using hyperbaric oxygen

HBO_2 therapeutic mechanisms of action are based on elevation both of the partial pressure of inspired O_2 and of the hydrostatic pressure. The latter mechanism contributes to determine the compression of all gas-filled spaces in the body (Boyle's law), and it is fundamental to allow an effective treatment of those conditions where gas bubbles are present in the body and cause the disease (e.g., intravascular embolism or decompression illness with intravascular or intra-tissue bubbles) [35, 36]. However, most patients treated with HBO_2 do not suffer from bubble-induced lesions, deriving their clinical improvements from the other mechanism of HBO_2 therapy: the elevated O_2 partial pressures achieved. High O_2 partial pressures so obtainable in various tissues lead to the increase in the production of reactive O_2 species (ROS) as well as of reactive nitrogen species (RNS), these last ones due to hyperoxia [37]. Controlled studies have already shown as the clinical efficacy from HBO_2 depends on modulation of intracellular transduction cascades, driving to synthesis of growth factors, promoting the wound healing, and ameliorating postischemic and post-inflammatory injuries [36].

The actual inability to establish which will be the correct dose of HBO_2 to administer in each case is still depending on the lack in Level 1 evidence [1, 11]; as a matter of fact, the current scientific literature does not yet allow a clear identification of the optimal treatment protocol.

Nevertheless, HBO_2 is positioned among the possible and feasible therapies which allow to provide a delay in undergoing hip arthroplasty surgery; it is a reasonable postulate that such therapy can show a beneficial effect without having the invasiveness of a surgical approach.

HBO_2 increases extracellular oxygen concentration and reduces cellular ischemia and edema by inducing vasoconstriction [38]. Studies have already reported radiographic improvement in FHN at stage I according to the Steinberg classification, as well as a better pain control, compliance, and range of motion (ROM) in FHN at Ficat stages I–II [36]. Amid the possible effects of HBO_2, there is a reduced bone marrow pressure, leading to a significant pain relief, and an increased oxygen delivery to ischemic cells, thus relieving compartment syndrome so to prevent a progression in a further necrosis, stimulating angiogenesis and oxygen-dependent cells, and enhancing osteoclast and osteoblast function for remodeling and repair. Moreover, HBO_2 is also able to stimulate the multipotent fibroblasts in the bone marrow with an additional aid in the osteogenesis process [37].

In FHN treatment HBO facilitates oxygenation of hypoxic tissue and reduces edema by creating a high concentration of dissolved oxygen and inducing vasoconstriction. This may explain the early pain relief noticed in patients treated with this modality; by saturating the extracellular fluid with diffused oxygen, HBO treatment will lead to a better oxygenation of the ischemic bone cells, independently of circulating hemoglobin and without the extra-energy requirement to provide for the dissociation of oxygen from hemoglobin. Late effects of HBO are bone resorption, revascularization, and osteogenesis [5, 36].

Yang et al. quantitatively evaluated the hemodynamic flow in animal models with steroid-induced FHN by using multi-slice CT perfusion imaging. Especially in the early stage, they assessed how HBO therapy resulted in regional blood flow improvement in the ischemic tissues. Additionally, they found high-grade new bone formation and a well-regenerated hematopoietic tissue [39]. Moreover, recent studies focusing among osteoblasts differentiation and suppression osteoclasts showed positive results due to hyperbaric oxygen treatment. In particular, HBO shifted the balance between bone formation and bone resorption promoting regeneration [40, 41].

5. Clinical presentation

An early detection of FHN is of paramount importance as clinical success of the therapy is closely related to the stage which the treatment started in [42]. There are several procedures capable to intercept a suspected FHN at the onset or eventual early stages of the disease:

at the present time, histological studies, scintigraphy, functional bone evaluation, radiography, magnetic resonance imaging (MRI), and computer-assisted tomography (CAT) are the most current diagnostic methods available. At an early stage, FHN is usually asymptomatic or characterized by slight pain radiating to the knee and/or ipsilateral buttock.

It may present with a limited range of hip movement as well as stabbing pain, especially during a forced intra-rotation. FHN should be considered if the patient feels pain in the hips and has no risk factors in his clinical history. In particular, plain radiographs can often appear as normal in the early stages of necrosis. Patients with a history of previous necrosis should be observed for bilateral FHN; this condition has been reported up to 70% of the observations [43].

Classification systems currently in use for FHN include the Ficat and Steinberg systems [15].

The Ficat classification substantially relies on standard radiographic presentations, where phase I shows normal images; phase II indicates a normal contour, with evidence of a bone remodeling; stage III is characterized by subchondral collapse or flattening of the femoral head; and phase IV indicates a narrowing of the joint space, with secondary degenerative changes in the acetabulum. The Ficat classification system is however based on radiographic imaging; therefore, the real size of the lesion cannot be quantified up to a more proper and accurate measure of the radiological appearance of the disease.

Steinberg expands the Ficat system into six stages, including quantification of involvement of the femoral head within stages I–VI, with three further subsets each: mild (less than 15% radiographic involvement of the head's articular surface), moderate (with a 15–30% involvement of the head's articular surface), and severe (greater than 30% involvement of the head's articular surface) stages.

Recently, the Association Research Circulation Osseous (ARCO) has recommended a third standardized classification system relying on an interpolated comparison of different procedure findings: radiographic, MRI, bone scan, and histologic findings [15]. Anyhow, not even this can eliminate completely the intrinsic operator-dependent variability, making Ficat and ARCO classification systems still not sufficiently reliable to assess FHN occurrence [44].

FHN is currently diagnosed by plain anterior-posterior and frog leg lateral radiographs of the hip, followed by MRI; this is considered the most accurate benchmark. Other existing tools for assessing the FHN presentation, such as venography, bone marrow pressure measurements, and core biopsy, are rarely used.

6. Clinical management of femoral head necrosis

Many therapeutic modalities have been proposed, and their effects were recently reviewed by Sen [45] and Zalavras and Lieberman [17].

Where untreated, FHN is a progressive disease process in affected hip showing an intact articular survival rates of less than 60% in 5 years; furthermore, the survival rate in stage III is less than 10% [10, 13].

Actual clinical evidence clearly demonstrates that HBO is able to lead to an extended duration of the survival rate of the affected hips:

- Reis et al. treated 12 patients with stage I ANFH, one daily HBO session, for a total of 100 HBO treatments. They reported that 81% of HBO-exposed patients returned to normal MRI vs. only 17% in the untreated group [46].
- A double-blind, randomized, controlled, prospective study evaluated hyperbaric oxygen therapy on a cohort of 20 patients with unilateral FHN (Ficat stage II) [5]. All patients were treated with either compressed oxygen or compressed air (HBA); each patient received 30 treatments of HBO or HBA for 6 weeks. After the initial 6-week treatment, the blind was broken: all HBA patients were then offered to undergo HBO treatment. From this point on, the study veers toward an observational design study. Range of motion (ROM), stabilometry, and pain were assessed at the beginning of the study and after 10, 20, and 30 treatments by a blinded physician. Resonance images were obtained at a pretreatment stage, at 12-month post-HBO, and at a final 7-year follow-up (**Figure 1**). There was a significant pain improvement after HBO, with significance after 20 treatments on average. ROM improved likewise during HBO, for all parameters, after 20–30 treatments. At 7-year follow-up, all patients remained substantially pain-free and none required hip arthroplasty; an almost complete radiographic healing of the osteonecrosis was observed in seven of nine hips. Hyperbaric oxygen therapy does appear to be a viable treatment modality in patients with Ficat II FHN [5].
- Koren et al. used HBO to treat 68 patients (78 joints) with stage I and II disease; these authors' HBO protocol involved breathing 100% oxygen at 2.0–2.4 ATA for 90 min, for a total of 20 treatments. They reported that 88% of the HBO treatment group had improvement on MRI and a 93% survival rate of the joints at 11.1 ± 5.1 year of follow-up of 54 patients (58 joints) [10].
- Recently, the long-term effect of HBO in 217 patients with stage I, II, and III ANFH has been investigated [47]. These results validated previous findings: HBO shows itself to be able to significantly improve hip condition, alleviate pain, and, more importantly, avoid hip surgery in most of patients presenting a stage II disease. Moreover, this study further shows the beneficial effects of HBO in stage III patients, where hip pain is significantly reduced in most patients, hip surgery is avoided in approximately half of the patients, and the obtained results are maintained for up to 4 years [47].

One of the first studies, proposed by Baixe and colleagues, affirmed that 20 HBO treatments were sufficient for pain reduction [48]. As previously reported, Camporesi and colleagues showed that after 20–30 treatments patients were substantially pain-free [5]. However, 20 HBO treatments are not sufficient for the complete hip healing.

Even though there are many evidences among beneficial effects of HBO, there is still no agreement on the number of HBO treatments required. The recent work by Bosco and colleagues generated a mean number of 83.3 ± 24.8 [47], while in the study by Koren et al., the average number of treatments was 78.3 ± 24.2: this in itself is remarkably close [10]. In other papers the number of treatments widely ranges from 20 to 120 [49].

http://dx.doi.org/10.5772/intechopen.75026

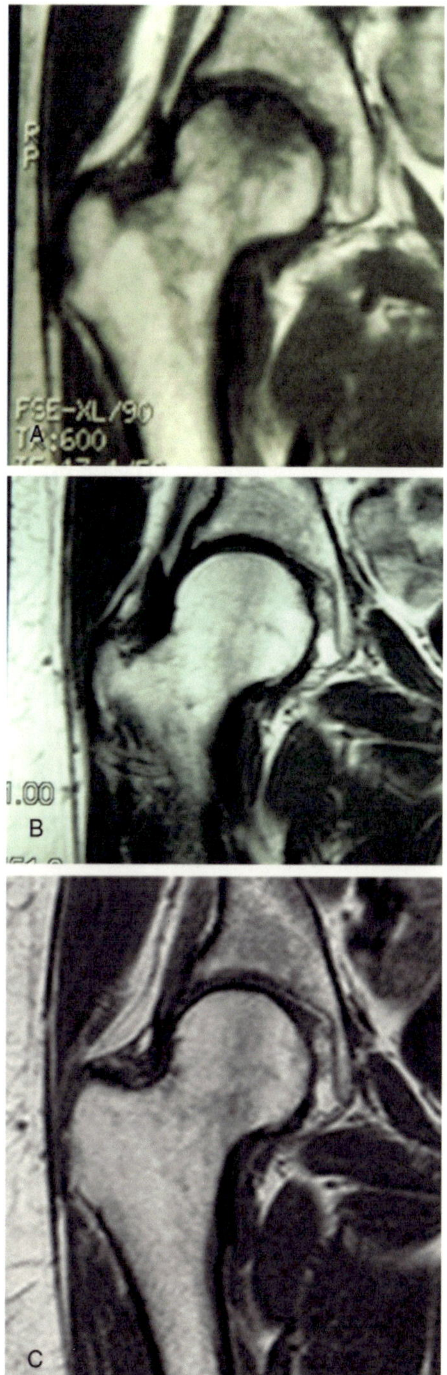

Figure 1. MRI pictures of a patient treated with HBO. (A) A pretreatment MRI exhibiting bone defect. (B) A twelve-month MRI showing near complete resolution of bone defect. (C) A seven-year follow-up MRI showing no change in bone defect [5].

A large number of sessions showed to be effective on pain relief and mobility improvement and avoided arthroplasty, in about 80% of cases. In particular, about 90% of Ficat I and II patients and half of Ficat III patients after HBOTs had no more need of surgery and all related complications for at least 4 years [47].

7. New perspectives

Despite the several clinical studies that support the benefits of HBOT in patients afflicted with osteonecrosis [1, 5], therapy is still not worldwide approved. This could be due to several factors including the apparent high number of HBO treatments necessary plus limited amount of clinical evidence for FHN, the majority of the evidence relies on ex vivo and in vitro studies, and the molecular mechanisms responsible for the regenerative responses of HBOT are still debatable. Thus, the underlying mechanism of action is still unclear.

A recent study investigated HBO upregulation on serum osteoprotegerin (OPG) and/or inhibition of osteoclast activation [50]. Twenty-three patients suffering from unilateral FHN at stage I, II, and III consented to the study: patients received standard HBOT; nineteen patients completed the study. Serum OPG levels were obtained at the beginning of HBOT (T_0), after 15 sessions (T_1), after 30 sessions (T_2), after a 30-day break (T_3), and at the end of our treatment protocol, after 60 sessions (T_4). Magnetic resonance imaging (MRI) was obtained at T_0 and about 1 year from the end of HBO treatments to compare pre-HBOT with post-HBOT lesion size.

The findings were:

- HBOT reduced pain symptoms in all patients.
- HBOT significantly reduced lesion size in all stage I and II patients and in 2 of 11 stage III patients.
- HBOT increased serum OPG levels, but receptor activator of nuclear factor kappa-B ligand (RANKL) levels did not change.

These evidences proposed an influence of HBO on the immune system and inflammatory processes. Indeed, one of the initial studies by Lukich et al. suggested an immunosuppressive effect of HBO therapy in patients suffering from rheumatoid arthritis [51]. Later, other studies reinforced these findings. Specifically, authors showed TNF-alpha and interleukin-1β (IL-1β) inhibition after HBO therapy in indomethacin-induced enteropathy and in chronic constriction injury-induced neuropathy [52, 53]. The following are some examples of tissue cytokine changes proposed after HBO.

IL-1β is a pro-inflammatory cytokine that responds to injury or infection by binding to the type-1 IL-1 receptor (IL-1R) and IL-1R accessory protein [54]. Although belonging to a structurally different cytokine class, IL-1 resembles many of the biological activities of TNF-α; IL-1 activation results in downstream activation of NF-kB and JNK [55, 56]. Fukushima et al. found that IL-1β has a stimulatory effect on osteoclast formation via increasing expression of RANKL [57]. IL-1β, like TNF-α and IL-6, is produced by stromal cells and monocytes. These cytokines can synergistically stimulate osteoclast differentiation leading to a net increase in RANKL activity and control their own expression [56].

IL-6 has been demonstrated to exhibit a dual effect on osteoclastic differentiation. During the inflammatory process, monocytes/macrophages produce IL-6, which can directly stimulate pre-osteoclast cells to be differentiated and activated [56]. In addition, IL-6 can stimulate stromal/osteoblastic cells to produce certain effectors, namely, IL-6, which will then promote osteoclastic differentiation [56]. Thus, there is a dual contribution, direct and indirect interaction, in which IL-6 can upregulate bone turnover. In vivo studies of IL-6 found that in transgenic mice with overexpressed IL-6 there is a greater bone turnover, reduced osteoblasts, and increased osteoclasts leading to osteopenia [58]. Correspondingly, IL-6-deficient mice displayed reduced osteoclasts and lower levels of bone erosion [59]. Kurokouchi and colleagues found TNF-α to increase the expression of IL-6 and ICAM-1 genes [60]. Hence, lower levels of TNF-α resulting from HBOT exposure could explain the reduction in IL-6. This effect, in summation with the synergistic effects of TNF-α, IL-6, and RANKL, could ultimately lead to decreased levels of osteoclastogenesis and, hence, greater resolution for the patient [56]. In the case of FHN, HBOT results in a decreased amount of circulating TNF-α. We propose the following mechanism: HBOT leads to reduced levels of TNF-α leading to decreased binding of TNF-α to the p55r type 1 receptor and thus decreased levels of NF-kB activation [56]. This reduction in RANKL would tip the balance of OPG/RANKL in the direction of osteoblast activation [50].

Understanding the HBOT's molecular mechanism of action remains the best approach in order to gain greater recognition for this treatment and to achieve earlier resolution for patients.

Author details

Gerardo Bosco[1]*, Alex Rizzato[1], Giuliano Vezzani[1], Vincenzo Zanon[1] and Enrico Camporesi[2]

*Address all correspondence to: gerardo.bosco@unipd.it

1 Master Level II in Diving and Hyperbaric Medicine and Physiological Lab, Department of Biomedical Sciences, University of Padova, Padova, Italy

2 Anesthesia, Tampa General Hospital, TEAM Health, Tampa, Florida, USA

References

[1] Camporesi E, Vezzani G, Zanon V, Manelli D, Enten G, Quartesan S, et al. Review on hyperbaric oxygen treatment in femoral head necrosis. Undersea & Hyperbaric Medicine. 2017;**44**(6):497-508

[2] Malizos KN, Karantanas AH, Varitimidis SE, Dailiana ZH, Bargiotas K, Maris T. Osteonecrosis of the femoral head: Etiology, imaging and treatment. European Journal of Radiology. 2007;**63**(1):16-28

[3] Parsons SJ, Steele N. Osteonecrosis of the femoral head: Part 1—Aetiology, pathogenesis, investigation, classification. Current Orthopaedics. 2007;**21**(6):457-463

[4] Babis GC, Sakellariou V, Parvizi J, Soucacos P. Osteonecrosis of the femoral head. Orthopedics. 2011;**34**(1):39

[5] Camporesi EM, Vezzani G, Bosco G, Mangar D, Bernasek TL. Hyperbaric oxygen therapy in femoral head necrosis. The Journal of Arthroplasty. 2010;**25**(6):118-123

[6] Shah KN, Racine J, Jones LC, Aaron RK. Pathophysiology and risk factors for osteonecrosis. Current Reviews in Musculoskeletal Medicine. 2015;**8**(3):201-209

[7] Steinberg M. Recent advances in the management of osteonecrosis of the hip. Seminars in Arthroplasty. 1998;(9):181-183

[8] Sun W, Shi Z, Gao F, Wang B, Li Z. The pathogenesis of multifocal osteonecrosis. Scientific Reports. 2016;**6**(1):29576

[9] Aaron R, Gray R. Osteonecrosis: Etiology, natural history, pathophysiology, and diagnosis. In: Callaghan JJ, Rosenberg AG, Rubash H, editors. The Adult Hip. Philadelphia: Lippincott Williams & Wilkins; 2007. pp. 465-476

[10] Koren L, Ginesin E, Melamed Y, Norman D, Levin D, Peled E. Hyperbaric oxygen for stage I and II femoral head osteonecrosis. Orthopedics. 2015;**38**(3):e200-e205

[11] Mathieu D, Marroni A, Kot J. Tenth European consensus conference on hyperbaric medicine: Preliminary report. Diving and Hyperbaric Medicine. 2016;**46**(2):122-123

[12] Clark J, Whelan HT. Oxygen toxicity. In: Kindwall EP, Wheland HT, editors. Hyperbaric medicine practice. Best Publishing Company; 1999. pp. 69-83

[13] Strauss M, Dvorak T, Melamed Y, Reis D. Femoral head necrosis and hyperbaric oxygen therapy. In: Flagsta AZ, editor. Hyperbaric Medicine Practice. North Palm Beach: Best Publishing Company; 2008. pp. 943-944

[14] Vezzani G, Bosco G, Camporesi EM. Hyperbaric oxygen treatment of avascular bone necrosis of the femoral head. In: Whelan HT, Kindwall EP, editors. Hyperbaric Medicine Practice. 4th ed. North Palm Beach: Best Publishing Company; 2017. pp. 955-974

[15] Amanatullah DF, Strauss EJ, Di Cesare PE. Current management options for osteonecrosis of the femoral head: Part 1, diagnosis and nonoperative management. The American Journal of Orthopedics. 2011 Sep;**40**(9):E186-E192

[16] Glueck CJ, Wang P, Freiberg RA. Osteonecrosis and thrombophilia: Pathophysiology, diagnosis, and treatment. In: Osteonecrosis of the Femoral Head. Cham: Springer International Publishing; 2017. pp. 3-17

[17] Zalavras CG, Lieberman JR. Osteonecrosis of the femoral head: Evaluation and treatment. The Journal of the American Academy of Orthopaedic Surgeons. 2014;**22**(7):455-464

[18] Israelite CL, Garino JP. Osteonecrosis of the hip. Seminars in Arthroplasty. 2005;**16**(1):27-32

[19] Graboń K, Paczesny Ł, Kruczyński J. Avascular necrosis of femoral condyles in a patient treated due to lymphoma. A case study. Ortopedia, Traumatologia, Rehabilitacja. 2017; **19**(5):469-480

[20] Shimizu J, Okazaki S, Nagoya S, Takahashi N, Kanaya K, Mizuo K, et al. Susceptibility of males, but not females to developing femoral head osteonecrosis in response to alcohol consumption. PLoS One. 2016;**11**(10):e0165490

[21] Fukushima W, Fujioka M, Kubo T, Tamakoshi A, Nagai M, Hirota Y. Nationwide epidemiologic survey of idiopathic osteonecrosis of the femoral head. Clinical Orthopaedics and Related Research. 2010;**468**(10):2715-2724

[22] Bauer TW, Stulberg BN. The histology of osteonecrosis and its distinction from histologic artifacts. In: Bone Circulation and Vascularization in Normal and Pathological Conditions. Boston, MA: Springer US; 1993. pp. 283-292

[23] Stulberg BN, Levine M, Bauer TW, Belhobek GH, Pflanze W, Feiglin DH, et al. Multimodality approach to osteonecrosis of the femoral head. Clinical Orthopaedics and Related Research. 1989;(240):181-193

[24] Brown TD, Baker KJ, Brand RA. Structural consequences of subchondral bone involvement in segmental osteonecrosis of the femoral head. Journal of Orthopaedic Research. 1992;**10**(1):79-87

[25] Kiaer T, Pedersen NW, Kristensen KD, Starklint H. Intra-osseous pressure and oxygen tension in avascular necrosis and osteoarthritis of the hip. Journal of Bone and Joint Surgery. British Volume (London). 1990;**72**(6):1023-1030

[26] Jarman MI, Lee K, Kanevsky A, Min S, Schlam I, Mahida C, et al. Case report: Primary osteonecrosis associated with thrombophilia-hypofibrinolysis and worsened by testosterone therapy. BMC Hematology. 2017;**17**(1):5

[27] Guo P, Gao F, Wang Y, Zhang Z, Sun W, Jiang B, et al. The use of anticoagulants for prevention and treatment of osteonecrosis of the femoral head: A systematic review. Medicine (Baltimore). 2017;**96**(16):e6646

[28] Cui Q, Wang GJ, Balian G. Steroid-induced adipogenesis in a pluripotential cell line from bone marrow. The Journal of Bone and Joint Surgery. American Volume. 1997 Jul; **79**(7):1054-1063

[29] Wang GJ, Cui Q, Balian G. The Nicolas Andry award. The pathogenesis and prevention of steroid-induced osteonecrosis. Clinical Orthopaedics and Related Research. 2000; **370**:295-310

[30] Pavićević A, Lakočević M, Popović M, Popović-Bijelić A, Daković M, Mojović M. Changes of the peripheral blood mononuclear cells membrane fluidity from type 1 Gaucher disease patients: An electron paramagnetic resonance study. Biological Chemistry. Jan 24, 2018 [Epub ahead of print]

[31] Linari S, Castaman G. Clinical manifestations and management of Gaucher disease. Clinical Cases in Mineral and Bone Metabolism. 2015;**12**(2):157-164

[32] Davidson J. Radiology of Dysbaric osteonecrosis. Journal of Clinical Pathology. 1972; **25**(11):1005-1006

[33] Uguen M, Pougnet R, Uguen A, Lodde B, Dewitte JD. Dysbaric osteonecrosis among professional divers: A literature review. Undersea & Hyperbaric Medicine. 2014;**41**(6): 579-587

[34] Sharareh B, Schwarzkopf R. Dysbaric osteonecrosis: A literature review of pathophysiology, clinical presentation, and management. Clinical Journal of Sport Medicine. 2015 Mar;**25**(2):153-161

[35] Vann RD, Butler FK, Mitchell SJ, Moon RE. Decompression illness. The Lancet. 2011; **377**(9760):153-164

[36] Camporesi EM, Bosco G. Mechanisms of action of hyperbaric oxygen therapy. Undersea & Hyperbaric Medicine. 2014;**41**(3):247-252

[37] Thom SR. Hyperbaric oxygen: Its mechanisms and efficacy. Plastic and Reconstructive Surgery. 2011;**127**(Suppl 1):131S-141S

[38] Bosco G, Yang Z, Nandi J, Wang J, Chen C, Camporesi EM. Effects of hyperbaric oxygen on glucose, lactate, glycerol and anti-oxidant enzymes in the skeletal muscle of rats during ischaemia and reperfusion. Clinical and Experimental Pharmacology & Physiology. 2007;**34**(1-2):70-76

[39] Yang J, Pan Z, Gu H, Li N, Qian X, Zhai R, et al. Quantitative study of therapeutic efficacy on early intervention of hyperbaric oxygen to model of steroid-induced avascular osteonecrosis of femoral head by multi-slice perfusion imaging. Zhonghua Yi Xue Za Zhi. 2008;**88**(45):3210-3216

[40] Al Hadi H, Smerdon GR, Fox SW. Hyperbaric oxygen therapy suppresses osteoclast formation and bone resorption. Journal of Orthopaedic Research. 2013;**31**(11):1839-1844

[41] Al Hadi H, Smerdon GR, Fox SW. Hyperbaric oxygen therapy accelerates osteoblast differentiation and promotes bone formation. Journal of Dentistry. 2015;**43**(3):382-388

[42] Hungerford D. Bone marrow pressure, venography and core decompression in ischemic necrosis of the femoral head. In: Riley L, editor. The Hip: Proceedings of the Seventh Open Scientific Meeting of the Hip Society. Saint Louis: CV Mosby; 1979. pp. 218-237

[43] Boettcher WG, Bonfiglio M, Hamilton HH, Sheets RF, Smith K. Non-traumatic necrosis of the femoral head. I. Relation of altered hemostasis to etiology. Journal of Bone & Joint Surgery. 1970;**52**(2):312-321

[44] Schmitt-Sody M, Kirchhoff C, Mayer W, Goebel M, Jansson V. Avascular necrosis of the femoral head: Inter- and intraobserver variations of Ficat and ARCO classifications. International Orthopaedics. 2008;**32**(3):283-287

[45] Sen RK. Management of avascular necrosis of femoral head at pre-collapse stage. Indian Journal of Orthopaedics. 2009;**43**(1):6-16

[46] Reis ND, Schwartz O, Militianu D, Ramon Y, Levin D, Norman D, et al. Hyperbaric oxygen therapy as a treatment for stage-I avascular necrosis of the femoral head. Journal of Bone and Joint Surgery. British Volume (London). 2003;**85**(3):371-375

[47] Vezzani G, Camporesi EM, Mangar D, Bernasek T, Yang Z, Quartesan S, et al. Bene cial e ect of hyperbaric oxygenation in avascular necrosis of the femoral head. Gazze a Medica Italiana Archivio per le Scienze Mediche. 2018;**3**(1):18-26

[48] Baixe J, Bidart J, Nicolini J. Treatment of osteonecrosis of the femoral head by hyperbaric oxygen. Bulletins: Medecine Subaquatique et Hyperbare. 1969;1:2

[49] Uzun G, Mutluoglu M, Ersen O, Yildiz S. Hyperbaric oxygen therapy in the treatment of osteonecrosis of the femoral head: A review of the current literature. Undersea and Hyperbaric Medicine. 2016;**43**(3):189-199

[50] Vezzani G, Quartesan S, Cancellara P, Camporesi E, Mangar D, Bernasek T, et al. Hyperbaric oxygen therapy modulates serum OPG/RANKL in femoral head necrosis patients. Journal of Enzyme Inhibition and Medicinal Chemistry. 2017;**32**(1):707-711

[51] Lukich VL, Poliakova LV, Sotnikova TI, Belokrinitskiĭ DV. Hyperbaric oxygenation in the comprehensive therapy of patients with rheumatoid arthritis (clinico-immunologic study). Fiziolohichnyi Zhurnal;**37**(5):55-60

[52] Yang Z, Nandi J, Wang J, Bosco G, Gregory M, Chung C, et al. Hyperbaric oxygenation ameliorates indomethacin-induced Enteropathy in rats by modulating TNF-α and IL-1β production. Digestive Diseases and Sciences. 2006;**51**(8):1426-1433

[53] Li F, Fang L, Huang S, Yang Z, Nandi J, Thomas S, et al. Hyperbaric oxygenation therapy alleviates chronic constrictive injury-induced neuropathic pain and reduces tumor necrosis factor-alpha production. Anesthesia and Analgesia. 2011;**113**(3):626-633

[54] Greenfeder SA, Nunes P, Kwee L, Labow M, Chizzonite RA, Ju G. Molecular cloning and characterization of a second subunit of the interleukin 1 receptor complex. The Journal of Biological Chemistry. 1995;**270**(23):13757-13765

[55] Baud V, Liu ZG, Bennett B, Suzuki N, Xia Y, Karin M. Signaling by proinflammatory cytokines: Oligomerization of TRAF2 and TRAF6 is sufficient for JNK and IKK activation and target gene induction via an amino-terminal effector domain. Genes & Development. 1999;**13**(10):1297-1308

[56] Steeve KT, Marc P, Sandrine T, Dominique H, Yannick F. IL-6, RANKL, TNF-alpha/IL-1: Interrelations in bone resorption pathophysiology. Cytokine & Growth Factor Reviews. 2004;**15**(1):49-60

[57] Fukushima H, Jimi E, Okamoto F, Motokawa W, Okabe K. IL-1-induced receptor activator of NF-κB ligand in human periodontal ligament cells involves ERK-dependent PGE2 production. Bone. 2005;**36**(2):267-275

[58] De Benedetti F, Rucci N, Del Fattore A, Peruzzi B, Paro R, Longo M, et al. Impaired skeletal development in interleukin-6–transgenic mice: A model for the impact of

chronic inflammation on the growing skeletal system. Arthritis and Rheumatism. 2006;**54**(11):3551-3563

[59] Ohshima S, Saeki Y, Mima T, Sasai M, Nishioka K, Nomura S, et al. Interleukin 6 plays a key role in the development of antigen-induced arthritis. Proceedings of the National Academy of Sciences. 1998;**95**(14):8222-8226

[60] Kurokouchi K, Kambe F, Yasukawa K, Izumi R, Ishiguro N, Iwata H, et al. TNF-α increases expression of IL-6 and ICAM-1 genes through activation of NF-κB in osteoblast-like ROS17/2.8 cells. Journal of Bone and Mineral Research. 1998;**13**(8):1290-1299

Chapter 3

Hyperbaric Oxygen Therapy in Traumatic Brain Injury: Cellular and Molecular Mechanisms

Sanja Pekovic, Sanja Dacic, Danijela Krstic,
Rada Jeremic, Marina Djelic and Predrag Brkic

Additional information is available at the end of the chapter

http://dx.doi.org/10.5772/intechopen.75025

Abstract

Traumatic brain injuries (TBI) are among the leading causes of death and chronic disability worldwide. TBI is a complex process encompassing primary injury to the brain tissue and cerebral vasculature induced by the initial impact, secondary injury, including cascade of subsequent neuroinflammatory processes, and regenerative responses with enhanced neurogenesis and angiogenesis. To date, there remains no approved pharmacological therapy that is able to prevent the secondary injury. Therefore, the development of safe and efficacious neuroprotective treatments currently represents the greatest unmet need in the management of TBI. Increasing number of experimental and clinical studies present convincing evidence that hyperbaric oxygen therapy (HBOT), as an adjunctive therapy, may be the suitable neurotherapeutic method for improving neurological outcome after TBI. Irrespective to treatment protocol HBOT appeared to alleviate the detrimental and neurotoxic effects of pathological sequel initiated by TBI and to stimulate endogenous reparative mechanisms. However, the exact mechanisms by which HBOT exerts its beneficial effects on recovery after brain injury are still deficient. In this review we will summarize up to date results of HBOT in experimental and clinical TBI and try to put more light on cellular and molecular mechanisms underlying beneficial effects of HBOT on functional recovery after brain injury.

Keywords: hyperbaric oxygen therapy, traumatic brain injury, neuroprotection, oxidant/antioxidant balance, oxidative stress, anti-apoptosis, anti-inflammation, neuronal plasticity, synaptogenesis, neurogenesis, angiogenesis

1. Introduction

Traumatic brain injuries (TBI) are one of the leading causes of death and chronic disability especially among the working population, and represent an important public health problem worldwide. Globally, about 10 million people are affected by TBI every year with projections that TBI will be one of the major causes of death and disability by the year 2020 [1]. Since TBI is a complex injury that encompasses a broad spectrum of symptoms and disabilities, the manifestations of head injury may be clinically very variable ranging from mild, to moderate or severe, depending on the extent and duration of damage to the brain. Many cognitive, physical and psychological skills can be affected, exerting a devastating impact on the patients and their family [2]. Over the years more than 30 phase III clinical trials failed emphasizing the urgent need for efficient treatment modalities and new directions in the future research to improve posttraumatic morbidity and mortality. Considering the complexity of TBI it is reasonable to assume that only combination of different treatment protocols could provide better prognosis for recovery to all forms of TBI [3]. In this view, hyperbaric oxygenation (HBO) or hyperbaric oxygen therapy (HBOT) appeared as an adjunctive therapy that may have the synergistic effect with other treatment protocols, suggesting that combining therapies with HBOT could provide better results than either alone [4]. According to definition given by the Undersea and Hyperbaric Medical Society (UHMS), hyperbaric medicine is a therapeutic approach in which a patient breathes 100% oxygen intermittently, while the pressure of the treatment chamber is higher than ambient (1 atmosphere absolute, 1 ATA = 101.3 kPa) [5–7]. In comparison to the normobaric conditions increased oxygen supply under hyperbaric conditions enables easier diffusion of oxygen into the injured tissue [8]. Accordingly, the HBOT can be used to obtain 100% saturation of hemoglobin and to significantly elevate the volume of physically dissolved oxygen fraction in blood plasma. This increased blood oxygen level then can penetrate to ischemic areas and perilesioned tissue more deeply than under normobaric conditions [9–11]. Thus, the HBOT has found its place, as the primary or adjuvant therapy in the treatment protocols for different clinical conditions [12, 13].

On the other hand, opinions about usage of HBOT as adjunctive therapy for the treatment of patients with brain injuries are still controversial [14–16]. In this way HBO is a very motivating therapeutic modality, which is known to produce oxidative stress by itself [17], but reduces oxidative stress when used in pathological conditions [18, 19]. The main concern in HBOT is oxidative stress and/or oxygen toxicity that can affect multiple organs. However, these side-effects are dependent on treatment parameters – pressure and duration of the treatment [20–23].

Substantial amount of evidences has been published indicating that HBOT can interfere with the processes that are following brain injury and moderate its consequences [14, 24–27]. Recent results of experimental and clinical studies and potential mechanisms of HBOT in TBI are reviewed by Wang et al. [28] and Hu et al. [7]. However, knowledge about the exact mechanisms by which HBOT exerts its beneficial effects is still deficient. Therefore, data presented in this chapter are meant to put more light on cellular and molecular mechanisms underlying neuroprotective effects of hyperbaric oxygenation after the brain injury.

2. Potential cellular and molecular mechanisms underlying HBOT

Increasing number of animal studies on HBOT in experimental TBI revealed a myriad of diverse mechanisms that may underlie neuroprotective effects of HBOT. Researchers suggested that many of these cellular and molecular mechanisms and signaling pathways work in parallel, or together, contributing to repair of the injured brain [6, 7, 23, 25, 28]. These mechanisms involve: (1) alleviation of secondary injury; (2) increasing of tissue oxygenation; (3) reducing of neurodegeneration; (4) decreasing of apoptosis; (5) regulation of oxidant/antioxidant status; (6) reduction of oxidative stress; (7) attenuation of reactive gliosis (microgliosis and astrogliosis) and glial scarring; (8) reducing of inflammation; (9) enhancement of neuronal plasticity; (10) promoting of synaptogenesis, neurogenesis and angiogenesis.

2.1. HBOT suppresses development of secondary brain damage

TBI involves primary and secondary injury. Primary injury occurs at the time of the impact and is the result of immediate mechanical damage of neural pathways followed by a permanent neuronal lost. The site of mechanical impact is called the "core". Surrounding regions consist of neuronal tissue that have not been directly affected by trauma and are often addressed to as "penumbra area". Neurons inside this zone are at risk due to a cascade of events, known as secondary injury that involves: impaired blood flow (limited or not at all), inflammation, development of edema, acidosis and hemorrhage, and the loss of most of their connections with the other neurons [11, 21, 22]. Secondary degeneration can also progress into the surrounding intact regions of the brain. Compromised blood flow and insufficient oxygen supply leads to tissue hypoxia and the resulting energy failure, which initiates a cascade of cellular events that culminate with neuronal cell apoptosis [23]. Thus, the consequence of secondary injury is degeneration of neurons that previously have not been exposed to trauma [29–31]. Most of the neurotherapeutic strategies are directed toward the containment of the secondary processes and the preservation and reactivation of the penumbra area and perilesioned region [30]. Cumulative evidence have proved that HBOT may reduce development of secondary brain damage and prevent neuronal apoptosis in animal models of TBI [32, 25], ischemic stroke [33–37], and hypoxia-ischemia [38–40], which was manifested by diminishing of brain infarction area and improvement of neurological deficits. Recently, Baratz-Goldstein et al. [41] demonstrated that both immediate (initiated 3 h post-injury) and delayed treatments with HBO (initiated 7 days post-injury) have a potential to prevent a neuronal loss in mouse model of moderate TBI.

2.2. HBOT reduces neuronal degeneration and prevents apoptosis after brain injury by regulation of oxidant/antioxidant status and reduction of oxidative stress

One of the main processes in this pathological cascade is oxidative stress that develops in the cells which have been exposed to trauma and in the cells at "penumbra area". Reactive oxygen species (ROS) are one of the products of oxidative stress [2] that are responsible for cellular damaging and apoptosis. The first line of the defense against ROS are enzymes located in mitochondria, such as manganese superoxide dismutase (SOD2) [42]. In our previous study, we have shown that repetitive HBOT influenced the pattern of SOD2 expression both on gene and protein level in cortical stab injury model (CSI) of TBI [43]. We applied HBO protocol of 60 min exposure to 100% oxygen at 2.5 ATA, once a day for 3 or 10 consecutive days. HBOT significantly increased mRNA levels of SOD2 at both time points compared to the corresponding lesioned group. Exposure to HBOT for 3 days down-regulated SOD2 protein levels in the injured cortex, while after 10 days of HBOT an up-regulation of SOD2 was observed. Using double-immunofluorescence staining we have demonstrated that HBOT attenuated SOD2 expression both in neuronal and astroglial cells surrounding the lesion site. Staining of the injured cortex with Fluoro-Jade®B (as a marker of degenerating neurons) revealed that HBOT significantly decreased the number of degenerating neurons in the injured cortex, and this effect was more pronounced after 10 consecutive HBOT. In according to this, we concluded that antioxidative and neuroprotective effect of HBOT is in part due to its influence on expression pattern of SOD2 [43].

In this chapter, using the cortical suction ablation (CSA) model of brain injury, described in our previous publications [44, 45], and the same HBOT protocol, we demonstrated that 10 repetitive HBOT altered activities of antioxidant enzymes and reduced lipid peroxidation, thereby preventing neuronal degeneration and apoptosis. Oxidant/antioxidant status in the injured cortex after HBOT is presented in **Figure 1**. HBOT significantly increased glutathione-peroxidase (GPX) activity in the injured cortex compared to all other groups. Injury markedly lowered the level of superoxide dismutase (SOD) activity, while HBOT returned SOD activity to almost control levels. The content of Malondialdehyde (MDA), which was used as an indicator of lipid peroxidation and reflects the membrane damage caused by ROS, was the highest in the tissue samples from injured cortex. HBOT initiated statistically significant reduction of MDA levels, pointing to preservation of membrane integrity. The similar trend of changes of MDA levels was determined in the serum indicating that serum concentrations of MDA may be used as a marker of degree of brain damage.

To evaluate the effect of HBOT on neurodegeneration/apoptosis we performed double-immunofluorescence staining: neurons undergoing degeneration were visualized with Fluoro-Jade®B, while NeuN (neuronal cell nuclei) was used as a marker of neuronal cell bodies. As it is shown in **Figure 2**, in the perilesioned cortex a huge number of neurons undergoing degeneration (**Figure 2A**, **E**) was significantly reduced after the HBOT (**Figure 2B**, **F**). Moreover, when the cortical sections from the injured (L) group were observed at higher magnification the formation of apoptotic bodies (**Figure 2G**, **I**, asterisks) in the neuronal nuclei was observed, indicating that they have entered into the process of apoptosis. On the contrary, in the sections from LHBO group the majority of neurons have healthy nuclei in which the nucleolus was clearly visible (**Figure 2H**, **J**, arrow heads). These results indicate that increased activities of antioxidant enzymes and reduction of lipid peroxidation underlies observed neuroprotective and anti-apoptotic effects of HBOT. Similarly, Li et al. [51], in the rat model of brain ischemia-reperfusion injury (IRI), have shown that HBO preconditioning lessened neuronal injury, reduced the level of MDA and increased the antioxidant activity of catalase (CAT) and SOD. They suggested that an up-regulation of the antioxidant enzyme activities after HBO preconditioning may play an important role in the generation of tolerance against IRI.

Maintaining proper mitochondrial function is essential for cellular function, since ROS are formed in mitochondria when energy metabolism is compromised. Niizuma and co-workers [52] demonstrated that mitochondrial dysfunction and oxidative stress may determine neuronal

http://dx.doi.org/10.5772/intechopen.75025

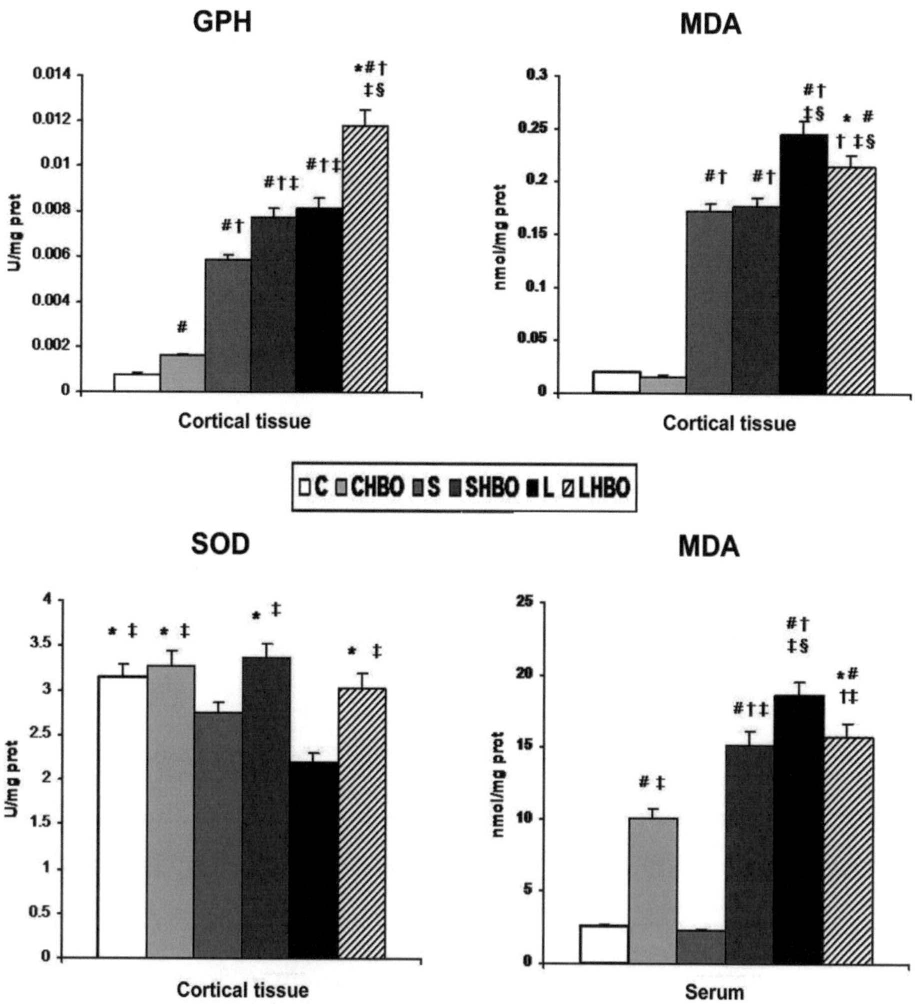

Figure 1. Effects of HBOT and cortical injury on the activities of antioxidant enzymes and lipid peroxidation in the injured cortex. Glutathione-peroxidase (GPX) activity is measured using coupled enzyme method by measuring the decrease of NADPH at 340 nm [46] and is expressed as unites per milligram of protein (U/mg). One unit (U) catalyzes the oxidation by H_2O_2 of 1.0 μmol of reduced glutathione to oxidized glutathione per minute. Total superoxide dismutase (SOD) activity is determined at room temperature according to the method of Misra and Fridovich [47], and is measured at 480 nm. One unit of SOD is defined as the amount of enzyme that inhibits the speed of oxidation of epinephrine for 50%. The results are expressed as U/mg of protein. Malondialdehyde (MDA) content is determined both in the injured cortex and serum. Thiobarbituric acid (TBA) reactive product MDA is used as an indicator of lipid peroxidation. MDA content is measured according to the method of Aruoma et al. [48] as described previously in Mladenovic et al. [49]. The absorbance of the organic phase is read at 532 nm. The values are expressed as nmol of MDA/mg of protein, using a standard curve of 1,1,3,3-tetramethoxypropane. Total protein was quantified according to Lowry's method [50] using bovine serum albumin as standard. Values are mean ± SD from $n \geq 4$ independent determinations performed in duplicate. Acronyms for the groups (n = 8 per group) are as follows: C – intact control, CHBO intact control subjected to the HBO protocol, S – sham surgery, SHBO sham control HBO group, L - injured group and LHBO - injured group subjected to the HBO protocol. Significant difference from corresponding group * $P < 0.05$ vs. L, # $P < 0.05$ vs. C, † $P < 0.05$ vs. CHBO, ‡ $P < 0.05$ vs. S, § $P < 0.05$ vs. SHBO.

death/survival after stroke and neurodegeneration. Therefore, a lot of studies have been conducting with purpose of finding out whether HBOT have a role in the preservation of mitochondrial function and integrity [25, 32, 53–55]. Palzur, Vlodavsky and their colleagues,

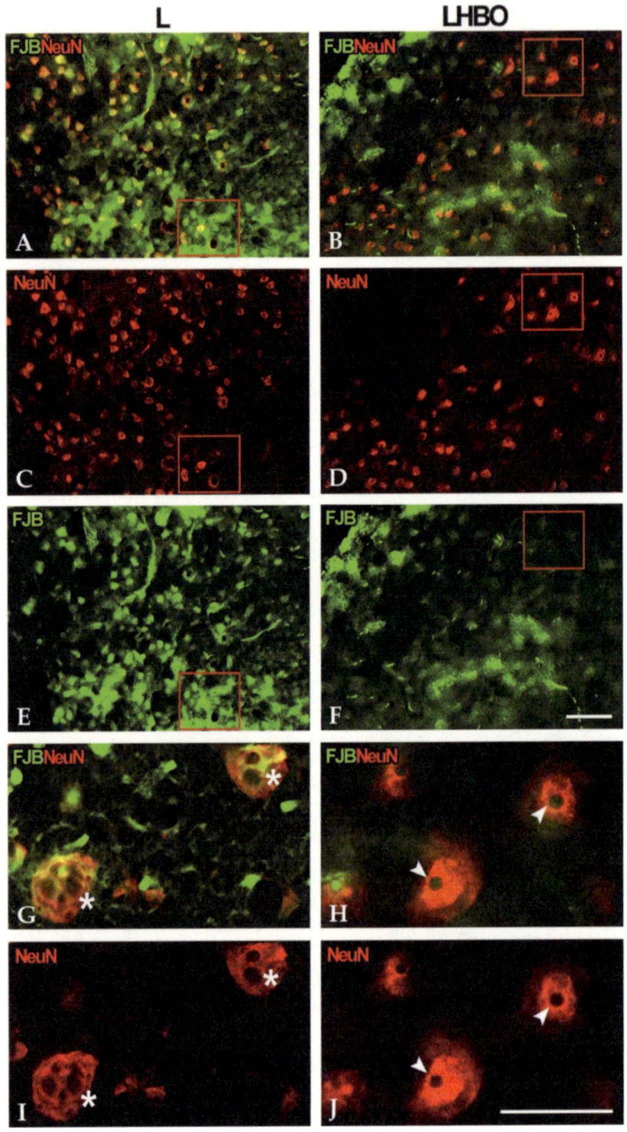

Figure 2. HBOT reduces neurodegeneration and prevents apoptosis in the injured cortex. Fluoro-jade®B staining (green) is performed in order to visualize neuronal cells undergoing degeneration and cell death, while NeuN (red) is used as a marker of neuronal cell bodies. Procedure for double-immunofluorescence staining was as described in Parabucki et al. [43]. Cortical sections were incubated with mouse anti-NeuN (1:200, Milipore, USA) and then with 0.0004% solution of Fluoro-Jade®B (FJB, Chemicon International, Temecula, CA, USA) dissolved in 0.1% acetic acid. The slides were examined with Carl Zeiss AxioVert microscope with AxioCam monochromatic camera (Zeiss, Goettingen, Germany), equipped with ApoTome software for optical sectioning. (**A, C, E**) A huge number of NeuN$^+$ neurons in the perilesioned cortex were co-stained with FJB (**A**, yellow fluorescence) indicating that they are undergoing neurodegeneration. Strikingly, when the cortical sections from the injured (L) group were observed at higher magnification, the formation of apoptotic bodies (**G, I**, asterisks) in the neuronal nuclei was observed, suggesting that they have entered into the process of apoptosis. (**B, D, F**) after 10 repetitive HBOT the number of NeuN$^+$/FJB$^+$ (**B**) and FJB$^+$ (**F**) neurons was negligible. Correspondingly, in the LHBO cortical sections the majority of neurons have healthy nuclei in which the nucleolus was clearly visible (**H, J**, arrow heads). Rectangles indicate where the high magnification images are taken from. Scale bars: (A-J) 50 μm.

http://dx.doi.org/10.5772/intechopen.75025

using cortical deformation model of TBI and the HBO protocol which consisted of two successive 45 min sessions at 2.8 ATA, have shown that increased concentrations of oxygen in the cells lead to preservation of mitochondrial integrity due to significant decrease of the loss of mitochondrial trans-membrane potential. Additionally, HBOT reduced the release of pro-apoptotic mediators Cytochrome C (Cyt C) and the Bcl-2-associated X protein (Bax) from mitochondria, and up-regulated the expression of anti-apoptotic protein Bcl-2 (B-cell lymphoma 2), consequently alleviating neuronal apoptosis in the injured brain tissue [56]. Zhou et al. [57] have emphasized that maintenance of mitochondrial function is one of the most important effects of HBOT.

TBI leads to the impairment of cerebral oxygen delivery and consumption [58]. So, the main problem is how to make cerebral hyperoxia, which is possible either under normobaric (NBH) or hyperbaric conditions. Clinical trials have shown that hyperbaric O2 has better effect than NBH on oxidative cerebral metabolism due to its ability to produce a brain tissue PO2 > or = 200 mm Hg, which represents a graduated effect [14].

Oxidative stress, and/or oxygen toxicity as unwanted side-effects of HBOT, as well as the fact that inhalation of pure oxygen at high pressures may lead to generation of ROS led researches to investigate which anti-oxidants can be used during HBO therapy. Studies have shown that hydrogen gas (H2) could be useful for this purpose. It alleviates oxygen toxicity due to reduction of hydroxyl radical levels [59]. Even, adding of inert gases, such as argon or xenon during HBO treatments can potentially make further improvement of cerebral lesions [60].

2.3. HBOT attenuates reactive microgliosis, astrogliosis and glial scarring after brain injury

After the injury astrocytes become rapidly activated during the process of "reactive astrogliosis" and accumulate around the lesion site, acting as a barrier that impedes neuroregeneration and neurite outgrowth, and isolates intact CNS tissue from secondary lesions [61, 62]. Proportionally to the severity of injury, they undergo cell proliferation, hypertrophy, increased expression of glial fibrillary acidic protein (GFAP) and vimentin, and exhibit an enhancement of immune-modulating capacities [2, 44, 63–66]. In our recently published paper [66] we have shown that repetitive HBOT attenuates reactive astrogliosis, prevent glial scar formation, and down-regulates GFAP and vimentin gene, protein and tissue expression in the perilesioned cortex. Similarly, Baratz-Goldstein et al. [41] demonstrated that both immediate and delayed HBOT have a potential to reduce reactive astrogliosis in mice model of TBI. Here, we reported that HBOT reduces reactive microgliosis around the lesion site as well (**Figure 3B**). Besides decreasing the number of activated microglia, HBOT also alters the morphology of activated microglia to more ramified, resting form (**Figure 3B** upper rectangle, **D** inset, **F** inset).

HBO-induced suppression of microgliosis and astrogliosis was reported to give an account to beneficial effects of HBO treatment in different rat models of TBI [41, 67, 68], cerebral ischemia [69], neuropathic and inflammatory pain [70, 71]. In contrast, Lee et al. [72] reported that prolonged HBOT may increase degree of gliosis indicating that longer oxygen cycling might help overcoming detrimental effects of gliosis and providing its beneficial effects.

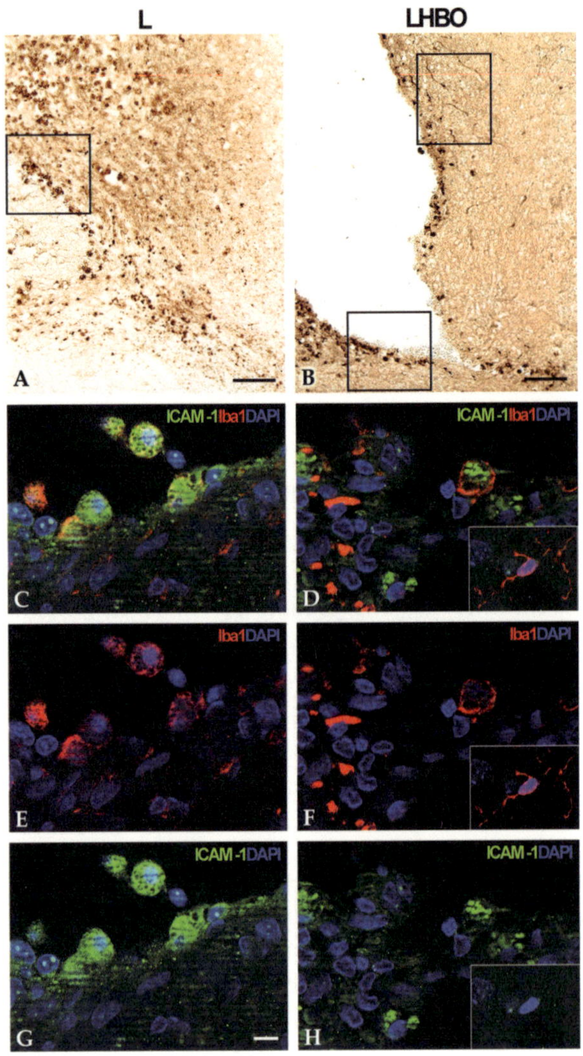

Figure 3. HBOT reduces reactive microgliosis in the perilesioned cortex and down-regulates ICAM-1 expression on microglial cells. (**A**) and (**B**) Effect of HBOT on reactive microgliosis in the injured cortex is determined using mouse anti-CD68 antibody (ED1, 1:100, Abcam, Cambridge, MA, USA) as a marker of activated microglia/macrophages. After using appropriate peroxidase linked secondary antibody (1:200, Santa Cruz Biotechnology, Santa Cruz, CA, USA), the products of immunoreactions were visualized with 3′3-diaminobenzidine (DAB, Dako, Glostrup, Denmark). Immunohistochemical and immunofluorescence staining was performed as described in Lavrnja et al. [66]. (**A**) after cortical injury a huge number of activated microglia/macrophages are seen around and within the lesion site. (**B**) HBOT (60 min exposure to 100% oxygen at 2.5 ATA) initiated daily for 10 consecutive days attenuated reactive microgliosis and alters morphology of activated microglia to more ramified, resting form (**B**, upper rectangle). (**C–H**) expression of ICAM-1 (green) on microglial cells stained with Iba1 (red) in cortices of injured (L) and injured group subjected to HBO protocol (LHBO) is visualized with immunofluorescence double-labeling. Cortical sections were incubated with goat anti-ICAM1 (1:100; Santa Cruz Biotechnology, Santa Cruz, CA, USA) and mouse anti-Iba1 (ionized calcium binding adaptor molecule 1, 1:500, Abcam, Cambridge, MA, USA) antibody, while nuclei were counterstained with DAPI (Invitrogen, Grand Island, NY, USA). All sections were photographed with Carl Zeiss Axiovert microscope with AxioCam monochromatic camera (Zeiss, Goettingen, Germany), equipped with ApoTome software for optical sectioning. (**C, E, G**) activated microglia characterized with round morphology showed up-regulation of ICAM-1 expression (**G**). (**D, F, H**) repetitive HBOT downregulated ICAM-1 expression on activated microglia within the lesion site. Microglial cells with ramified morphology (insets to **D** and **F**) do not express ICAM-1 (insets to **D** and **H**). Rectangles indicate where the high magnification images are taken from. Scale bars: (**A, B**) 50 μm (**C–H**) 5 μm.

2.4. HBOT prevents spreading of the neuroinflammation in the injured tissue

Inflammation is an important part of the pathophysiology of TBI and has a pivotal role in the extent of neuronal injury and repair. It is postulated that the initiation, progression and resolution of inflammation in TBI is multifaceted. These processes involve migration, recruitment and infiltration of leukocytes following blood-brain barrier (BBB) disruption and activation of resident immune cells of the CNS (microglia, astrocytes). Microglia and astrocytes then acquire immunological function and secrete inflammatory mediators such as pro- and anti-inflammatory cytokines, chemokines, adhesion molecules, complement factors, ROS and other factors [58, 73, 74]. The accumulation of neutrophils around the site of injury and their infiltration into the injured brain area is crucial for the initiation and progression of inflammation and the extent of secondary brain damage since they may release free oxygen and nitrogen radicals and pro-inflammatory cytokines [54, 58]. Neutrophils initially attach to vascular endothelium via binding to the endothelial intercellular adhesion molecules (ICAMs). In our previously mentioned paper [66] we have demonstrated injury-induced increase of gene and tissue expression of ICAM-1 (Intercellular Adhesion Molecule-1, CD54), an adhesion molecule that is important for trans-endothelial migration of neutrophils and propagation of inflammation [75, 76]. Using double- immunofluorescence staining we demonstrated its localization on various type of cells (astrocytes, vascular endothelium, neurons, activated microglia/macrophages and neutrophils), around the blood vessels, and in the proximity and within the lesion site. Ten successive treatments with HBO significantly decreased ICAM-1 mRNA expression returning it to control levels, while increased ICAM-1 immunoreactivity around the lesion site was diminished [66]. Herein, using double-immunofluorescence staining we have shown that HBOT reduced expression of ICAM-1 on activated microglia within the lesion site (**Figure 3H**). Furthermore, HBOT increased number of ramified/resting microglia in the perilesioned cortex (**Figure 3B**, upper rectangle). Interestingly, they do not express ICAM-1(**Figure 3H**, inset). These data indicate that HBOT by reducing ICAM-1 expression and targeting the passage of immune cells through the BBB via inhibition of cell adhesion molecules may contribute to dampen the neuroinflammatory response to TBI. Several studies also have shown that HBOT reduces the expression of ICAM-1 and adhesion of neutrophils to the endothelium, which is correlated with improved neurological outcome [54, 77–80].

CD40 ligand (CD40L, also termed CD154, or GP39) and its counter receptor CD40 (a membrane protein that belongs to the tumor necrosis factor (TNF) receptor family) are well-known regulators of pro-inflammatory and immune responses in the CNS [81], and are members of CD40/CD40L/ICAM-1 deleterious cascade of events after TBI. Given that CD40/CD40L dyad fosters neuroinflammation, it is suggested that CD40/CD40L interaction may be involved in modulating the outcome from injuries of the brain [82–84]. Accordingly, strategies aimed at suppressing CD40/CD40L/ICAM-1 expression may attenuate inflammation and neuronal damage after TBI, which will ultimately be of benefit in recovery [85]. In our recent paper [66] we have for the first time shown that HBOT prevents injury-induced up-regulation of expression of CD40 and its ligand CD40L on microglia/macrophages, neutrophils, cortical neurons and reactive astrocytes. These results indicate that repetitive HBOT, by limiting expression of inflammatory mediators, supports formation of more permissive environment for repair and regeneration.

Data of many studies has been shown that HBO suppress various mediators of inflammation [54, 67, 86, 87] indicating that the decreased brain edema, blood-brain barrier leakage, cell apoptosis and improved neurological outcome are closely related to the inhibitory effect of HBOT on inflammation after TBI [7]. During the early stage of TBI, effect of HBOT in reducing inflammation was achieved by increasing anti-inflammatory cytokine interleukin-10 (IL-10) and transforming growth factor-β1 (TGF-β1) expression, decreasing of the RNA and protein levels of caspase-3, interleukin-8 (IL-8), interleukin-6 (IL-6), tumor necrosis factor-α (TNF-α), macrophage inflammatory protein-2 (MIP-2), monocyte chemoattractant protein-1 (MCP-1) and transforming growth-interacting factor (TGIF), as well as via reduction of the expression of matrix metalloproteinase-9 (MMP9) [28, 54, 67, 68, 88–90]. Recently, Geng et al. [91] demonstrated that HBOT suppressed protein expression of inflammasome components and reduced the levels of interleukin-1β (IL-1β), interleukin-18 (IL-18) and high-mobility group box 1 (HMGB1) protein in the injured brain tissues and serum. Based on these results authors assumed that HBOT may diminish the inflammatory response after TBI by inhibiting the activation of inflammasome signaling. Latest results of Meng et al. [86] showed that HBOT significantly increased the expression of nuclear factor (erythroid-derived 2)- related factor 2 (Nrf2) and heme oxygenase-1, and inhibited the expression of Toll-like receptor 4 and nuclear factor-kappa B in a rat TBI model [87]. Furthermore, HBOT decreases expression of nNOS, eNOS and iNOS (neuronal, endothelial and inducible nitric oxide synthases) mRNA in the cortex after acute traumatic cerebral injury [92].

2.5. HBOT improves neurofunctional recovery of the injured brain by enhancing neuronal plasticity and synaptogenesis

Growing number of studies have reported that, irrespective to diversity of protocols, HBO therapy applied after TBI improved neurological status including motor and cognitive function, as well as learning and memory abilities, indicating that the best prognosis is achieved by earlier and continuous HBO treatment [11, 41, 45, 57, 67, 88, 93]. On the other hand, Baratz-Goldstein et al. [41] demonstrated that delayed treatment with HBO (initiated 7 days post-injury) also lead to improvement in learning abilities in mice model of moderate TBI. Additionally, in their recent publication Lim et al. [90] suggested that HBO treatment may ameliorate TBI-induced depression-like behavior in rats.

In our previously published paper [45] we have demonstrated that HBOT improves recovery of locomotor performances and sensorimotor integration after cortical injury in rats by enhancing neuroplastic responses and promoting synaptogenesis. Using growth-associated protein 43 (GAP43) and synaptophysin (SYP) as markers of axonal sprouting and synaptogenesis, respectively, we were the first to demonstrate that HBOT induces over-expression of GAP43 and SYP in the neurons surrounding the injury site. Given that an increase in GAP43 and SYP expression occurs concomitantly with improvement of locomotor abilities, we suggested that mechanisms underlying HBOT action involve promoting of axonal sprouting and the formation of new functional synaptic circuits. This implies that axonal reorganization and synapse remodeling contribute to observed functional recovery. Recent results of Zhang et al. [93] that HBOT-induced increase of GAP43 and synaptophysin expression underlies observed enhancement of learning abilities in the controlled cortical impact (CCI) model of rat brain injury confirmed our assumptions. Furthermore, Chen and Chen [94] detected

HBOT-induced enhancement of SYP expression after hypoxia-ischemia and proposed that the induction of synaptic plasticity and reducing of the ultrastructural damage may underlie rehabilitation mechanisms of HBOT.

2.6. HBOT promotes neurogenesis and angiogenesis after TBI

Nowadays, stem cells are in the center of attention. Stimulation of neurogenesis after HBOT and influence of stem cells mobilization on motor and cognitive performances is demonstrated in numerous studies [67, 95–97]. Thus, Shandley et al. [97] showed that cognitive improvement observed after treatment with HBO in patients with mild to moderate TBI is correlated with stem cell mobilization. Based on these findings they hypothesized that stem cells, mobilized by HBOT treatment, are recruited to repair damaged neuronal tissue. Yang et al. [98] and Wang et al. [99] reported that HBOT promotes the migration and differentiation of endogenous neural stem cells (NSCs) in neonatal rats with hypoxic-ischemic (HI) brain damage. Authors have shown that after HBOT, an increase in newly generated neurons, oligodendrocytes and remyelination was observed in the HI group treated with HBO compared to the untreated HI rats. Further, it was suggested that HBOT-stimulated proliferation of NSCs protects the learning and memory ability of the HI rats [100]. In our recent preliminary reports [101, 102] we also noticed that HBOT when applied after brain injury promoted endogenous NSCs to migrate to the site of injury and differentiate into mature neurons, contributing to improved neurofunctional recovery of the injured brain. Moreover, we demonstrated that HBOT alters morphology of neuronal precursors to more matured morphology [102].

Mu et al. [103] suggested that activation of several signaling pathways and transcription factors (Wnt, hypoxia-inducible factors - HIFs, and cAMP response element-binding - CREB) play an important role in HBOT-induced neurogenesis. Furthermore, it was assumed that endogenous neurogenesis, enhanced by application of delayed HBO in the late-chronic phase of stroke, is possibly mediated by ROS/HIF-1α/β-catenin pathway [96].

Interestingly, combining of HBOT with bone marrow stem cells (BMSCs) transplantation showed synergistic effect and had favorable influence in improving rehabilitation after rat spinal cord injury [104]. The same combination of HBOT and BMSCs transplantation proved to be more effective for repair of cognitive and neurological functions after TBI than monotherapy [105]. Similarly, long course of HBO treatments (for 3 weeks) promote the mobilization and migration of BMSCs to ischemic brain, stimulate expression of trophic factors and neurogenesis, and help in neuronal repair after ischemic stroke [72].

Besides neurogenesis HBOT may improve the outcome of TBI by stimulating angiogenesis [67, 95, 106, 107]. Using brain perfusion imaging, Tal et al. [106] demonstrated that 60 daily HBOT sessions stimulate cerebral angiogenesis in post-TBI patients, which induced significant improvement in the global cognitive scores. These data strongly suggest that one of the ways in which HBOT can induce neuroplasticity is angiogenesis. Given that HBOT was initiated 6 months to 27 years after the injury, obtained results imply that HBOT may improve perfusion to the chronic damaged brain tissue even months to years after the injury. Recent results of the same group [107] showed that in addition to the increased cerebral blood flow and volume, HBOT improved both white and gray microstructures pointing to regeneration of nerve fibers. These micro structural changes correlate with the significant improvement in the memory, executive functions, information processing speed and global cognitive scores.

3. Conclusions

HBOT has been used as a primary or adjunctive therapy over the last 50 years, both in experimental and clinical studies. However, despite the decades of extensive research the entire spectrum of HBOT action is still not completely understood, although many mechanisms of its action have been proposed. Therefore, in this systematic review we elaborate the cellular and molecular mechanisms of HBOT actions. Based on the presented data it may be concluded that improved tissue oxygenation and cellular metabolism, anti-inflammation, anti-apoptosis, as well as intensifying of neuroplastic responses, promoting of synaptogenesis, neurogenesis and angiogenesis may constitute the multiple and complementary mechanisms underlying HBOT-induced neuroprotection. In addition, reduction of lipid peroxidation and up-regulation of antioxidant enzymes are among the mechanisms involved in the action of HBO. In that way, HBOT diminishes imbalance between oxidants and anti-oxidants that occurs after brain injury, and contributes to the maintenance of pro−/antioxidant homeostasis. Furthermore, HBOT effectively attenuates reactive astrogliosis and microgliosis, prevents tissue-damaging effects of neutrophils and suppresses formation of glial scar. Accordingly, by alleviating glia-mediated inflammatory response and limiting production of inflammatory mediators HBOT fosters formation of more permissive environment for tissue repair, allowing the recovery of impaired brain functions. Overall, although results clearly suggest the validity of HBO therapy for the treatment of TBI, the underlying mechanism still needs to be studied in depth.

Acknowledgements

This work was supported by the Ministry of Education, Science and Technological Development of the Republic of Serbia, Grant III 41014. The authors would like to thank the Center for Hyperbaric Medicine, Belgrade, Serbia for their continuous support.

Conflict of interest

The authors declare that there is no conflict of interests regarding the publication of this paper.

Authors' contribution

SP performed surgery and wrote the paper; SD was responsible for tissue preparation, immunohistochemistry and immunofluorescence; DK carried out the enzyme and lipid peroxidation assays; RJ contributed substantially to the study by literature search and writing of the manuscript; PB carried out the HBOT and with MDj provided critical revision of the manuscript. All authors read and approved the final manuscript.

Author details

Sanja Pekovic[1]*, Sanja Dacic[2], Danijela Krstic[3], Rada Jeremic[4], Marina Djelic[4] and Predrag Brkic[4]

*Address all correspondence to: spekovic@ibiss.bg.ac.rs

1 Department of Neurobiology, Institute for Biological Research "Sinisa Stankovic", University of Belgrade, Belgrade, Serbia

2 Institute of Physiology and Biochemistry, Faculty of Biology, University of Belgrade, Belgrade, Serbia

3 Institute of Medical Chemistry, Faculty of Medicine, University of Belgrade, Belgrade, Serbia

4 Institute of Medical Physiology "Richard Burian", Faculty of Medicine, University of Belgrade, Belgrade, Serbia

References

[1] Hyder AA, Wunderlich CA, Puvanachandra P, Gururaj G, Kobusingye OC. The impact of traumatic brain injuries: A global perspective. NeuroRehabilitation. 2007;**22**(5):341-353

[2] Pekovic S, Subasic S, Nedeljkovic N, Bjelobaba I, Filipovic R, Milenkovic I, et al. Molecular basis of brain injury and repair. In: Ruzdijic S, Rakic LJ, editors. Neurobiological Studies – From Genes to Behaviour. Kerala, India: Research Signpost; 2006. pp. 143-165

[3] Margulies S, Hicks R. Combination therapies for traumatic brain injury: Prospective considerations. Journal of Neurotrauma. 2009;**26**(6):925-939. DOI: 10.1089/neu.2008.0794

[4] Michalski D, Küppers-Tiedt L, Weise C, Laignel F, Härtig W, Raviolo M, et al. Long-term functional and neurological outcome after simultaneous treatment with tissue-plasminogen activator and hyperbaric oxygen in early phase of embolic stroke in rats. Brain Research. 2009;**15, 1303**:161-168. DOI: 10.1016/j.brainres.2009.09.038

[5] Feldmeier JJ, editor. Hyperbaric Oxygen Therapy: 2003 Committee Report, Rev. Ed. Kensington (MD): Undersea and Hyperbaric Medical Society, Inc.; 2003. p. 137

[6] Brkic DP, Pekovic MS, Krstic ZD, Jovanovic ST. Hyperbaric oxygenation as an adjuvant therapy for traumatic brain injury: A review of literature. Periodicum Biologorum. 2014;**116**(1):29-36

[7] Hu Q, Manaenko A, Xu T, Guo Z, Tang J, Zhang J. Hyperbaric oxygen therapy for traumatic brain injury: Bench-to-bedside. Medical Gas Research. 2016;**6**(2):102-110. DOI: 10.4103/2045-9912.184720

[8] Gjedde A. The pathways of oxygen in brain. I. Delivery and metabolism of oxygen. Advances in Experimental Medicine and Biology. 2005;**566**:269-275. DOI: 10.1007/0-387-26206-7_36

[9] Daugherty WP, Levasseur JE, Sun D, Rockswold GL, Bullock MR. Effects of hyperbaric oxygen therapy on cerebral oxygenation and mitochondrial function following moderate lateral fluid-percussion injury in rats. Journal of Neurosurgery. 2004;**101**(3):499-504. DOI: 10.3171/jns.2004.101.3.0499

[10] Calvert JW, Cahill J, Zhang JH. Hyperbaric oxygen and cerebral physiology. Neurological Research. 2007;**29**(2):132-141. DOI: 10.1179/016164107X174156

[11] Wang GH, Zhang XG, Jiang ZL, Li X, Peng LL, Li YC, et al. Neuroprotective effects of hyperbaric oxygen treatment on traumatic brain injury in the rat. Journal of Neurotrauma. 2010;**27**(9):1733-1743. DOI: 10.1089/neu.2009.1175

[12] Kindwall EP. Uses of hyperbaric oxygen therapy in the 1990s. Cleveland Clinic Journal of Medicine. 1992;**59**(5):517-528

[13] Schaub E, Pellegrini M, Pugin D. Carbon monoxide poisoning: An update for 2009. Revue Médicale Suisse. 2009;**5**(213):1606-1609

[14] Rockswold SB, Rockswold GL, Zaun DA, Zhang X, Cerra CE, Bergman TA, et al. A prospective, randomized clinical trial to compare the effect of hyperbaric to normobaric hyperoxia on cerebral metabolism, intracranial pressure, and oxygen toxicity in severe traumatic brain injury. Journal of Neurosurgery. 2010;**112**(5):1080-1094. DOI: 10.3171/2009.7.JNS09363

[15] Rockswold SB, Rockswold GL, Zaun DA, Liu J. A prospective, randomized phase II clinical trial to evaluate the effect of combined hyperbaric and normobaric hyperoxia on cerebral metabolism, intracranial pressure, oxygen toxicity, and clinical outcome in severe traumatic brain injury. Journal of Neurosurgery. 2013;**118**(6):1317-1328. DOI: 10.3171/2013.2.JNS121468

[16] Bennett MH, Trytko B, Jonker B. Hyperbaric oxygen therapy for the adjunctive treatment of traumatic brain injury. Cochrane Database of Systematic Reviews. 2012;**12**:CD004609. DOI: 10.1002/14651858.CD004609.pub3

[17] Thom SR. Oxidative stress is fundamental to hyperbaric oxygen therapy. Journal of Applied Physiology (1985). 2009;**106**(3):988-995. DOI: 10.1152/japplphysiol.91004.2008

[18] Ozden TA, Uzun H, Bohloli M, Toklu AS, Paksoy M, Simsek G, et al. The effects of hyperbaric oxygen treatment on oxidant and antioxidants levels during liver regeneration in rats. The Tohoku Journal of Experimental Medicine. 2004;**203**(4):253-265

[19] Oter S, Korkmaz A, Topal T, Ozcan O, Sadir S, Ozler M, et al. Correlation between hyperbaric oxygen exposure pressures and oxidative parameters in rat lung, brain, and erythrocytes. Clinical Biochemistry. 2005;**38**(8):706-711. DOI: 10.1016/j.clinbiochem.2005.04.005

[20] Benedetti S, Lamorgese A, Piersantelli M, Pagliarani S, Benvenuti F, Canestrari F. Oxidative stress and antioxidant status in patients undergoing prolonged exposure to hyperbaric oxygen. Clinical Biochemistry. 2004;**37**(4):312-317. DOI: 10.1016/j.clinbiochem.2003.12.001

[21] Smerz RW. Incidence of oxygen toxicity during the treatment of dysbarism. Undersea & Hyperbaric Medicine. 2004;**31**(2):199-202

[22] Rockswold SB, Rockswold GL, Defillo A. Hyperbaric oxygen in traumatic brain injury. Neurological Research. 2007;**29**(2):162-172. DOI: 10.1179/016164107X181798

[23] Bitterman H. Bench-to-bedside review: Oxygen as a drug. Critical Care. 2009;**13**(1):205. DOI: 10.1186/cc7151

[24] Niklas A, Brock D, Schober R, Schulz A, Schneider D. Continuous measurements of cerebral tissue oxygen pressure during hyperbaric oxygenation--HBO effects on brain edema and necrosis after severe brain trauma in rabbits. Journal of the Neurological Sciences. 2004;**219**(1-2):77-82. DOI: 10.1016/j.jns.2003.12.013

[25] Palzur E, Vlodavsky E, Mulla H, Arieli R, Feinsod M, Soustiel JF. Hyperbaric oxygen therapy for reduction of secondary brain damage in head injury: An animal model of brain contusion. Journal of Neurotrauma. 2004;**21**(1):41-48. DOI: 10.1089/089771504772695931

[26] Lin JW, Tsai JT, Lee LM, Lin CM, Hung CC, Hung KS, et al. Effect of hyperbaric oxygen on patients with traumatic brain injury. Acta Neurochirurgica. Supplement. 2008;**101**:145-149

[27] Fischer BR, Speckmann EJ, Greiner C, Gorji A, Wölfer J, Wassmann H. Hyperbaric oxygen in neurosurgery. Acta Neurochirurgica. 2009;**151**(4):415-418. DOI: 10.1007/s00701-009-0228-2

[28] Wang Y, Chen D, Chen G. Hyperbaric oxygen therapy applied research in traumatic brain injury: From mechanisms to clinical investigation. Medical Gas Research. 2014;**4**(4):18. DOI: 10.1186/2045-9912-4-18

[29] Eriskat J, Plesnila N, Stoffel M, Baethmann A. Assessment of regional cortical blood flow following traumatic lesion of the brain. Acta Neurochirurgica. Supplement. 1997;**70**:94-95

[30] Thomale UW, Schaser K, Kroppenstedt SN, Unterberg AW, Stover JF. Cortical hypoperfusion precedes hyperperfusion following controlled cortical impact injury. Acta Neurochirurgica. Supplement. 2002;**81**:229-231

[31] Zauner A, Daugherty WP, Bullock MR, Warner DS. Brain oxygenation and energy metabolism: Part I-biological function and pathophysiology. Neurosurgery. 2002;**51**(2):289-301

[32] Palzur E, Zaaroor M, Vlodavsky E, Milman F, Soustiel JF. Neuroprotective effect of hyperbaric oxygen therapy in brain injury is mediated by preservation of mitochondrial membrane properties. Brain Research. 2008;**1221**:126-133

[33] Zhou JG, Liu JC, Fang YQ. Effect of hyperbaric oxygen on the expression of proteins Bcl-2 and Bax in the gerbil hippocampus CA1 following forebrain ischemia reperfusion. Zhongguo Ying Yong Sheng Li Xue Za Zhi. 2000;**16**(4):298-301

[34] Yin D, Zhou C, Kusaka I, Calvert JW, Parent AD, Nanda A, et al. Inhibition of apoptosis by hyperbaric oxygen in a rat focal cerebral ischemic model. Journal of Cerebral Blood Flow and Metabolism. 2003;**23**(7):855-864. DOI: 10.1097/01.WCB.0000073946.29308.55

[35] Li Y, Zhou C, Calvert JW, Colohan AR, Zhang JH. Multiple effects of hyperbaric oxygen on the expression of HIF-1 alpha and apoptotic genes in a global ischemia-hypotension rat model. Experimental Neurology. 2005;**191**(1):198-210. DOI: 10.1016/j.expneurol.2004.08.036

[36] Lou M, Ding MP, Wen SQ. Effect of hyperbaric oxygenation treatment on the apoptotic cell death pathway after transient focal cerebral ischemia. Zhongguo Ying Yong Sheng Li Xue Za Zhi. 2006;**22**(1):1-5

[37] Peng Z, Xiao P, Guo H, Liu Q. Effect of early hyperbaric oxygen on neuronal apoptosis and learning and memory of cerebral ischemia-reperfusion injury in rats. Zhong Nan Da Xue Xue Bao. Yi Xue Ban. 2009;**34**(6):468-475

[38] Calvert JW, Yin W, Patel M, Badr A, Mychaskiw G, Parent AD, et al. Hyperbaric oxygenation prevented brain injury induced by hypoxia-ischemia in a neonatal rat model. Brain Research. 2002;**951**(1):1-8

[39] Calvert JW, Zhou C, Nanda A, Zhang JH. Effect of hyperbaric oxygen on apoptosis in neonatal hypoxia-ischemia rat model. Journal of Applied Physiology (1985). 2003; **95**(5):2072-2080. DOI: 10.1152/japplphysiol.00630.2003

[40] Liu XH, Yan H, Xu M, Zhao YL, Li LM, Zhou XH, et al. Hyperbaric oxygenation reduces long-term brain injury and ameliorates behavioural function by suppression of apoptosis in a rat model of neonatal hypoxia-ischemia. Neurochemistry International. 2013; **62**(7):922-930. DOI: 10.1016/j.neuint.2013.03.004

[41] Baratz-Goldstein R, Toussia-Cohen S, Elpaz A, Rubovitch V, Pick CG. Immediate and delayed hyperbaric oxygen therapy as a neuroprotective treatment for traumatic brain injury in mice. Molecular and Cellular Neurosciences. 2017;**83**:74-82. DOI: 10.1016/j.mcn.2017.06.004

[42] Bidmon HJ, Kato K, Schleicher A, Witte OW, Zilles K. Transient increase of manganese-superoxide dismutase in remote brain areas after focal photothrombotic cortical lesion. Stroke. 1998;**29**(1):203-210

[43] Parabucki AB, Bozić ID, Bjelobaba IM, Lavrnja IC, Brkić PD, Jovanović TS, et al. Hyperbaric oxygenation alters temporal expression pattern of superoxide dismutase 2 after cortical stab injury in rats. Croatian Medical Journal. 2012;**53**(6):586-597

[44] Peković S, Filipović R, Subasić S, Lavrnja I, Stojkov D, Nedeljković N, et al. Down-regulation of glial scarring after brain injury: The effect of purine nucleoside analogue ribavirin. Annals of the New York Academy of Sciences. 2005;**1048**:296-310. DOI: 10.1196/annals.1342.027

[45] Brkic P, Stojiljkovic M, Jovanovic T, Dacic S, Lavrnja I, Savic D, et al. Hyperbaric oxygenation improves locomotor ability by enhancing neuroplastic responses after cortical ablation in rats. Brain Injury. 2012;**26**(10):1273-1284. DOI: 10.3109/02699052.2012.667593

[46] Wendel A. Enzymatic Basis of Detoxication. Vol. 1. NY: Academic Press; 1980. p. 333

[47] Misra HP, Fridovich I. The role of superoxide anion in the autoxidation of epinephrine and a simple assay for superoxide dismutase. The Journal of Biological Chemistry. 1972;**247**(10):3170-3175

[48] Aruoma OI, Halliwell B, Laughton MJ, Quinlan GJ, Gutteridge JM. The mechanism of initiation of lipid peroxidation. Evidence against a requirement for an iron (II)-iron (III) complex. Biochemical Journal. 1989;**258**(2):617-620

[49] Mladenović D, Krstić D, Colović M, Radosavljević T, Rasić-Marković A, Hrncić D, et al. Different sensitivity of various brain structures to thioacetamde-induced lipid peroxidation. Medicinal Chemistry. 2012;**8**(1):52-58

[50] Lowry OH, Rosebrough NJ, Farr AL, Randall RJ. Protein measurement with the Folin phenol reagent. The Journal of Biological Chemistry. 1951;**193**(1):265-275

[51] Li J, Liu W, Ding S, Xu W, Guan Y, Zhang JH, et al. Hyperbaric oxygen preconditioning induces tolerance against brain ischemia-reperfusion injury by upregulation of antioxidant enzymes in rats. Brain Research. 2008;**1210**:223-229. DOI: 10.1016/j.brainres.2008.03.007

[52] Niizuma K, Endo H, Chan PH. Oxidative stress and mitochondrial dysfunction as determinants of ischemic neuronal death and survival. Journal of Neurochemistry. 2009;**109**(1):133-138. DOI: 10.1111/j.1471-4159.2009.05897.x

[53] Vlodavsky E, Palzur E, Feinsod M, Soustiel JF. Evaluation of the apoptosis-related proteins of the BCL-2 family in the traumatic penumbra area of the rat model of cerebral contusion, treated by hyperbaric oxygen therapy: A quantitative immunohistochemical study. Acta Neuropathologica. 2005;**110**(2):120-126. DOI: 10.1007/s00401-004-0946-8

[54] Vlodavsky E, Palzur E, Soustiel JF. Hyperbaric oxygen therapy reduces neuroinflammation and expression of matrix metalloproteinase-9 in the rat model of traumatic brain injury. Neuropathology and Applied Neurobiology. 2006;**32**(1):40-50. DOI: 10.1111/j.1365-2990.2005.00698.x

[55] Soustiel JF, Palzur E, Vlodavsky E, Veenman L, Gavish M. The effect of oxygenation level on cerebral post-traumatic apoptotsis is modulated by the 18-kDa translocator protein (also known as peripheral-type benzodiazepine receptor) in a rat model of cortical contusion. Neuropathology and Applied Neurobiology. 2008;**34**(4):412-423. DOI: 10.1111/j.1365-2990.2007.00906.x

[56] Liu Z, Jiao QF, You C, Che YJ, Effect SFZ. Of hyperbaric oxygen on cytochrome C, Bcl-2 and Bax expression after experimental traumatic brain injury in rats. Chinese Journal of Traumatology. 2006;**9**(3):168-174

[57] Zhou Z, Daugherty WP, Sun D, Levasseur JE, Altememi N, Hamm RJ, et al. Protection of mitochondrial function and improvement in cognitive recovery in rats treated with hyperbaric oxygen following lateral fluid-percussion injury. Journal of Neurosurgery. 2007;**106**(4):687-694. DOI: 10.3171/jns.2007.106.4.687

[58] Werner C, Engelhard K. Pathophysiology of traumatic brain injury. British Journal of Anaesthesia. 2007;**99**(1):4-9. DOI: 10.1093/bja/aem131

[59] Yu J, Yu Q, Liu Y, Zhang R, Xue L. Hydrogen gas alleviates oxygen toxicity by reducing hydroxyl radical levels in PC12 cells. PLoS One. 2017;**12**(3):e0173645. DOI: 10.1371/journal.pone.0173645

[60] Chhor V, Canini F, De Rudnicki S, Dahmani S, Gressens P, Constantin P. Hyperbaric oxygen therapy and inert gases in cerebral ischemia and traumatic brain injury. Annales Françaises d'Anesthèsie et de Rèanimation. 2013;**32**(12):863-871. DOI: 10.1016/j.annfar.2013.09.005

[61] Silver J, Miller JH. Regeneration beyond the glial scar. Nature Reviews. Neuroscience. 2004;**5**(2):146-156. DOI: 10.1038/nrn1326

[62] Sofroniew MV. Molecular dissection of reactive astrogliosis and glial scar formation. Trends in Neurosciences. 2009;**32**(12):638-647. DOI: 10.1016/j.tins.2009.08.002

[63] Calingasan NY, Erdely HA, Altar CA. Identification of CD40 ligand in Alzheimer's disease and in animal models of Alzheimer's disease and brain injury. Neurobiology of Aging. 2002;**23**(1):31-39

[64] Pekny M, Wilhelmsson U, Bogestål YR, Pekna M. The role of astrocytes and complement system in neural plasticity. International Review of Neurobiology. 2007;**82**:95-111. DOI: 10.1016/S0074-7742(07)82005-8

[65] Sofroniew MV, Vinters HV. Astrocytes: Biology and pathology. Acta Neuropathologica. 2010;**119**(1):7-35. DOI: 10.1007/s00401-009-0619-8

[66] Lavrnja I, Parabucki A, Brkic P, Jovanovic T, Dacic S, Savic D, et al. Repetitive hyperbaric oxygenation attenuates reactive astrogliosis and suppresses expression of inflammatory mediators in the rat model of brain injury. Mediators of Inflammation. 2015;**2015**:498405

[67] Lin KC, Niu KC, Tsai KJ, Kuo JR, Wang LC, Chio CC, et al. Attenuating inflammation but stimulating both angiogenesis and neurogenesis using hyperbaric oxygen in rats with traumatic brain injury. Journal of Trauma and Acute Care Surgery. 2012;**72**(3):650-659. DOI: 10.1097/TA.0b013e31823c575f

[68] Lim SW, Wang CC, Wang YH, Chio CC, Niu KC, Kuo JR. Microglial activation induced by traumatic brain injury is suppressed by postinjury treatment with hyperbaric oxygen therapy. The Journal of Surgical Research. 2013;**184**(2):1076-1084. DOI: 10.1016/j.jss.2013.04.070

[69] Günther A, Küppers-Tiedt L, Schneider PM, Kunert I, Berrouschot J, Schneider D, et al. Reduced infarct volume and differential effects on glial cell activation after hyperbaric oxygen treatment in rat permanent focal cerebral ischaemia. The European Journal of Neuroscience. 2005;**21**(11):3189-3194. DOI: 10.1111/j.1460-9568.2005.04151.x

[70] Hui J, Zhang ZJ, Zhang X, Shen Y, Gao YJ. Repetitive hyperbaric oxygen treatment attenuates complete Freund's adjuvant-induced pain and reduces glia-mediated neuroinflammation in the spinal cord. The Journal of Pain. 2013;**14**(7):747-758. DOI: 10.1016/j.jpain.2013.02.003

[71] Zhao BS, Meng LX, Ding YY, Cao YY. Hyperbaric oxygen treatment produces an antinociceptive response phase and inhibits astrocyte activation and inflammatory response in a rat model of neuropathic pain. Journal of Molecular Neuroscience. 2014;**53**(2):251-261. DOI: 10.1007/s12031-013-0213-3

[72] Lee YS, Chio CC, Chang CP, Wang LC, Chiang PM, Niu KC, et al. Long course hyperbaric oxygen stimulates neurogenesis and attenuates inflammation after ischemic stroke. Mediators of Inflammation. 2013;**2013**:512978. DOI: 10.1155/2013/512978

[73] Morganti-Kossmann MC, Satgunaseelan L, Bye N, Kossmann T. Modulation of immune response by head injury. Injury. 2007;**38**(12):1392-1400. DOI: 10.1016/j.injury.2007.10.005

[74] Hellewell SC, Morganti-Kossmann MC. Guilty molecules, guilty minds? The conflicting roles of the innate immune response to traumatic brain injury. Mediators of Inflammation. 2012;**2012**:356494. DOI: 10.1155/2012/356494

[75] Benveniste EN, Nguyen VT, Wesemann DR. Molecular regulation of CD40 gene expression in macrophages and microglia. Brain, Behavior, and Immunity. 2004;**18**(1):7-12

[76] Yilmaz G, Granger DN. Leukocyte recruitment and ischemic brain injury. Neuromolecular Medicine. 2010;**12**(2):193-204. DOI: 10.1007/s12017-009-8074-1

[77] Buras JA, Stahl GL, Svoboda KK, Reenstra WR. Hyperbaric oxygen downregulates ICAM-1 expression induced by hypoxia and hypoglycemia: The role of NOS. American Journal of Physiology. Cell Physiology. 2000;**278**(2):C292-C302

[78] Atochin DN, Fisher D, Demchenko IT, Thom SR. Neutrophil sequestration and the effect of hyperbaric oxygen in a rat model of temporary middle cerebral artery occlusion. Undersea & Hyperbaric Medicine. 2000;**27**(4):185-190

[79] Miljkovic-Lolic M, Silbergleit R, Fiskum G, Rosenthal RE. Neuroprotective effects of hyperbaric oxygen treatment in experimental focal cerebral ischemia are associated with reduced brain leukocyte myeloperoxidase activity. Brain Research. 2003;**971**(1):90-94

[80] Helms AK, Whelan HT, Torbey MT. Hyperbaric oxygen therapy of cerebral ischemia. Cerebrovascular Diseases. 2005;**20**(6):417-426. DOI: 10.1159/000088979

[81] Chen K, Huang J, Gong W, Zhang L, Yu P, Wang JM. CD40/CD40L dyad in the inflammatory and immune responses in the central nervous system. Cellular & Molecular Immunology. 2006;**3**(3):163-169

[82] Calingasan NY, Erdely HA, Altar CA. Identification of CD40 ligand in Alzheimer's disease and in animal models of Alzheimer's disease and brain injury. Neurobiology of Aging. 2002;**23**(1):31-39

[83] Garlichs CD, Kozina S, Fateh-Moghadam S, Handschu R, Tomandl B, Stumpf C, et al. Upregulation of CD40-CD40 ligand (CD154) in patients with acute cerebral ischemia. Stroke. 2003;**34**(6):1412-1418. DOI: 10.1161/01.STR.0000074032.64049.47

[84] Ishikawa M, Vowinkel T, Stokes KY, Arumugam TV, Yilmaz G, Nanda A, et al. CD40/CD40 ligand signaling in mouse cerebral microvasculature after focal ischemia/reperfusion. Circulation. 2005;**111**(13):1690-1696. DOI: 10.1161/01.CIR.0000160349.42665.0C

[85] Zhang B, Wu T, Chen M, Zhou Y, Yi D, Guo R. The CD40/CD40L system: A new therapeutic target for disease. Immunology Letters. 2013;**153**(1-2):58-61. DOI: 10.1016/j.imlet.2013.07.005

[86] Meng XE, Zhang Y, Li N, Fan DF, Yang C, Li H, et al. Effects of hyperbaric oxygen on the Nrf2 signaling pathway in secondary injury following traumatic brain injury. Genetics and Molecular Research. 2016a;**15**(1). DOI: 10.4238/gmr.15016933

[87] Meng XE, Zhang Y, Li N, Fan DF, Yang C, Li H, et al. Hyperbaric oxygen alleviates secondary brain injury after trauma through inhibition of TLR4/NF-κB Signaling pathway. Medical Science Monitor. 2016b;**22**:284-288

[88] Chen X, Duan XS, Xu LJ, Zhao JJ, She ZF, Chen WW, et al. Interleukin-10 mediates the neuroprotection of hyperbaric oxygen therapy against traumatic brain injury in mice. Neuroscience. 2014;**266**:235-243. DOI: 10.1016/j.neuroscience.2013.11.036

[89] Wee HY, Lim SW, Chio CC, Niu KC, Wang CC, Kuo JR. Hyperbaric oxygen effects on neuronal apoptosis associations in a traumatic brain injury rat model. The Journal of Surgical Research. 2015;**197**(2):382-389. DOI: 10.1016/j.jss.2015.04.052

[90] Lim SW, Sung KC, Shiue YL, Wang CC, Chio CC, Kuo JR. Hyperbaric oxygen effects on depression-like behaviour and Neuroinflammation in traumatic brain injury rats. World Neurosurgery. 2017;**100**:128-137. DOI: 10.1016/j.wneu.2016.12.118

[91] Geng F, Ma Y, Xing T, Zhuang X, Zhu J, Yao L. Effects of hyperbaric oxygen therapy on Inflammasome signalling after traumatic brain injury. Neuroimmunomodulation. 2016;**23**(2):122-129. DOI: 10.1159/000445689

[92] Zhou JG, Fang YQ, Liu CY, Zhou YQ, Ji YF, Liu JC. Effect of hyperbaric oxygen on the expression of nitric oxide synthase mRNA in cortex after acute traumatic cerebral injury. Zhongguo Ying Yong Sheng Li Xue Za Zhi. 2012;**28**(1):38-41

[93] Zhang X, Wang X, Sun X, Sun X, Zhang Y, Zhang H. Differences in cognitive function of rats with traumatic brain injuries following hyperbaric oxygen therapy. Medical Science Monitor. 2016;**22**:2608-2615

[94] Chen J, Chen YH. Effects of hyperbaric oxygen on synaptic ultrastructure and synaptophysin expression in hippocampus of neonatal rats with hypoxic-ischemic brain damage. Zhonghua Er Ke Za Zhi. 2010;**48**(3):199-203

[95] Zhang T, Yang QW, Wang SN, Wang JZ, Wang Q, Wang Y, et al. Hyperbaric oxygen therapy improves neurogenesis and brain blood supply in piriform cortex in rats with vascular dementia. Brain Injury. 2010;**24**(11):1350-1357. DOI: 10.3109/02699052.2010.504525

[96] Hu Q, Liang X, Chen D, Chen Y, Doycheva D, Tang J, et al. Delayed hyperbaric oxygen therapy promotes neurogenesis through reactive oxygen species/hypoxia-inducible factor-1α/β-catenin pathway in middle cerebral artery occlusion rats. Stroke. 2014; **45**(6):1807-1814. DOI: 10.1161/STROKEAHA.114.005116

[97] Shandley S, Wolf EG, Schubert-Kappan CM, Baugh LM, Richards MF, Prye J. Increased circulating stem cells and better cognitive performance in traumatic brain injury subjects following hyperbaric oxygen therapy. Undersea & Hyperbaric Medicine. 2017; **44**(3):257-269

[98] Yang YJ, Wang XL, Yu XH, Wang X, Xie M, Liu CT. Hyperbaric oxygen induces endogenous neural stem cells to proliferate and differentiate in hypoxic-ischemic brain damage in neonatal rats. Undersea & Hyperbaric Medicine. 2008;**35**(2):113-129

[99] Wang XL, Yang YJ, Xie M, Yu XH, Wang QH. Hyperbaric oxygen promotes the migration and differentiation of endogenous neural stem cells in neonatal rats with hypoxic-ischemic brain damage. Zhongguo Dang Dai Er Ke Za Zhi. 2009;**11**(9):749-752

[100] Wei L, Wang J, Cao Y, Ren Q, Zhao L, Li X, et al. Hyperbaric oxygenation promotes neural stem cell proliferation and protects the learning and memory ability in neonatal hypoxic-ischemic brain damage. International Journal of Clinical and Experimental Pathology. 2015;**8**(2):1752-1759. DOI: PMC4396307

[101] Brkic P, Dacic S, Jeremic R, Jovanovic T, Pekovic S. The efect of hyperbaric oxygenation on neurogenesis after brain injury in adult rats. Alessandro Marroni, Maja Medić, Mariana Sedlar and Minjon Zarić Milanović, editors. IX International Congress on Hyperbaric Medicine; May 11th-14th; Belgrade, Serbia. Belgrade: Centre for Hyperbaric Medicine; 2017. p. 26

[102] Jeremic R, Dacic S, Brkic P, Djelic M, Jovanovic T, Pekovic S. Hyperbaric oxygenation enhances neurogenesis after injury to adult rat brain. Selma Kanazir and Ivana Bjelobaba, editors. 7th Congress of Serbian Neuroscience with international participation; October 25th–27th; Belgrade, Serbia. Belgrade: Serbian Neuroscience Society, Serbian Ministry of Education, Science and Technological development, Institute for Biological Research "Sinisa Stankovic", University of Belgrade; 2017. p. 84. ISBN: 978-86-917255-1-8

[103] Mu J, Krafft PR, Zhang JH. Hyperbaric oxygen therapy promotes neurogenesis: Where do we stand? Medical Gas Research. 2011;**1**(1):14. DOI: 10.1186/2045-9912-1-14

[104] Geng CK, Cao HH, Ying X, Yu HL. Effect of mesenchymal stem cells transplantation combining with hyperbaric oxygen therapy on rehabilitation of rat spinal cord injury. Asian Pacific Journal of Tropical Medicine. 2015;**8**(6):468-473. DOI: 10.1016/j.apjtm.2015.05.001

[105] Zhou HX, Liu ZG, Liu XJ, Chen QX. Umbilical cord-derived mesenchymal stem cell transplantation combined with hyperbaric oxygen treatment for repair of traumatic brain injury. Neural Regeneration Research. 2016;**11**(1):107-113. DOI: 10.4103/1673-5374.175054

[106] Tal S, Hadanny A, Berkovitz N, Sasson E, Ben-Jacob E, Efrati S. Hyperbaric oxygen may induce angiogenesis in patients suffering from prolonged post-concussion syndrome due to traumatic brain injury. Restorative Neurology and Neuroscience. 2015;**33**(6):943-951. DOI: 10.3233/RNN-15058

[107] Tal S, Hadanny A, Sasson E, Suzin G, Efrati S. Hyperbaric oxygen therapy can induce angiogenesis and regeneration of nerve Fibers in traumatic brain injury patients. Frontiers in Human Neuroscience. 2017;**11**:508. DOI: 10.3389/fnhum.2017.00508

Chapter 4

Microcirculation and Hyperbaric Oxygen Treatment

Fethi Gul, Omer Faruk Boran and Reyhan Arslantas

Additional information is available at the end of the chapter

http://dx.doi.org/10.5772/intechopen.75609

Abstract

The microcirculation is anatomical and consists of arterioles, capillaries, and venules that perform metabolic requirements and oxygen distribution to the tissues. During physiological or pathological stress, it balances between the oxygen delivery and the demand. This delicate balance can play an important role in the progression of critical illnesses and has a role in the development of organ dysfunction. Reduced microvascular perfusion is seen in many diseases, and hyperbaric oxygen treatment (HBOT) has potentially beneficial effects on the microcirculatory environment. It has been shown that HBOT improves microcirculation independent from systemic hemodynamic parameters, which is a key therapeutic target in the critically ill patient. HBOT is emerging as an adjunct to traditional surgery and antibiotic therapy for the special kinds of problematic wounds or purpura fulminans, which are caused by meningococcal sepsis. HBOT also can increase oxygen supply to the ischemic tissue to reduce the extent of irreversible tissue damage in ischemic stroke, femoral head necrosis, diabetic foot ulcer, and carbon monoxide intoxication. In this chapter, we aim to describe microcirculation with its monitoring systems and to show the effectiveness of HBOT in different clinical settings, which are related to microcirculatory dysfunction.

Keywords: hyperbaric oxygen, microcirculatory dysfunction, perfusion, critical illness

1. Microcirculation physiology

The area of the circulation system where the metabolic requirements of tissues are met is called microcirculation. In other words, this is the point at which the arterial system and venous system join.

As a result of 6–8 branches occurring in the arterial structure entering a tissue, the width of the interior lumen reduces to 10–15 μm, and this structure is called an arteriole. The wall structures of arterioles continue with metarterioles within the continuous surrounding smooth muscle, and capillary veins form from metarterioles. At the point where the capillaries emerge from the metarterioles, smooth muscle tissue forms a sphincter-like structure at the capillary entrance. Capillary structures continue to form venules. Venules have the larger diameter compared to arterioles though they have less muscle tissue. However, less muscle tissue causes low pressure within the venule and ensures severe contractile force (**Figure 1**).

The total wall thickness of capillary structures is 0.5 μm. Shaped elements in the blood can only pass through by friction along the wall of the 9-μm lumen. There are openings of 6–7 nm width between the endothelial cells of the capillaries called fenestrations. These structures form 1/1000 of the total endothelial surface area but are areas where the transfer of water and water-soluble material occurs. These fenestrations may differ from organ to organ. These gaps are very narrow in the brain, while in the kidneys broad intervals ensure the necessary width for glomerular filtration of water and solutes [1].

Capillaries are not continuously open structures. The number of open capillaries varies depending on the requirements of the tissue, and here the most important stimulus is the oxygen

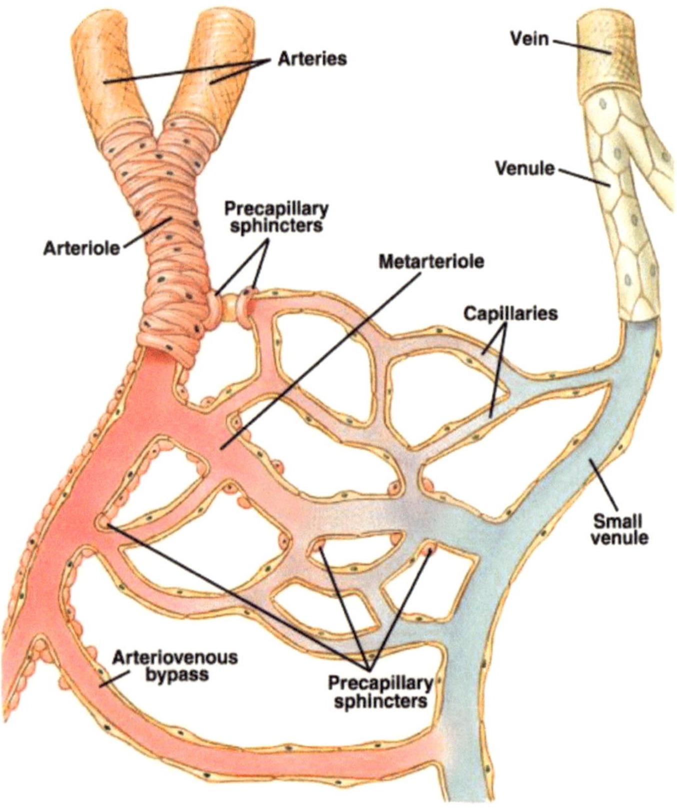

Figure 1. The area of the circulation system.

http://dx.doi.org/10.5772/intechopen.75609

requirement of the tissue. The precapillary sphincter found at the junction of the metarterioles with capillaries plays a role in the opening of closed capillaries and closure of open capillaries, and this local control is called vasomotion [2].

There may be nearly 12 l of fluid found in the interstitial area. This cavity found between cells is kept open by collagen fibres. Proteoglycans appear to be like a brush for the interstitium. Due to proteoglycans found in the interstitial fluid, it has a gel consistency. Water and electrolytes may rapidly diffuse within the gel. Free fluid is only found in collagen fibres and at cell boundaries in the interstitial area.

The size of exchange areas for material transfer between compartments in the microcirculatory environment is directly related to the transfer amounts. Additionally, other effective factors are fixed transfer, the presence of membrane carriers, channel-dependent transport, barrier permeability, and soluble material transfer [3].

According to Fick's first law, the solute transfer from a membrane only occurs in situations with concentration differences until concentration balance is achieved [4].

$$J_s = P_d S[\Delta C]$$

where J_s is the solute flow rate, P_d is the diffusion permeability constant, and ΔC is the concentration difference

$$P_d = \frac{D_f}{\Delta x'}$$

where D_f is the free diffusion constant, and Δx is the barrier thickness.

According to Fick's second law, the amount of diffusion is linked to the thickness of the membrane, the surface area over which diffusion occurs, molecular mass and size.

$$\frac{dn}{dt} = -DA\frac{\Delta C}{\Delta X}$$

About 97% of oxygen is bound to haemoglobin in blood and passes into tissues according to the Fick law. Oxygen presentation to tissues is dependent on the cardiac output and arterial oxygen content. Formula of arterial oxygen content is the sum of the multiplication of oxygen saturation, blood haemoglobin level and Hüfner number (amount of oxygen carried if haemoglobin is fully filled) with the multiplication of partial oxygen pressure by 0.003. There is 100 mmHg oxygen pressure at the arterial tip at the 1 atmospheric pressure while at the pressure of 3 atmospheres with 100% oxygen it increases according to the Henry law and reaches to the 2000 mmHg. Tissue oxygen pressure reaches from 55 to 500 mmHg at this point. At 1 atmosphere pressure, there is 3 ml per litre of free oxygen, and this amount reaches 60 ml where the tissues fulfil their needs without using haemoglobin-bound oxygen [5].

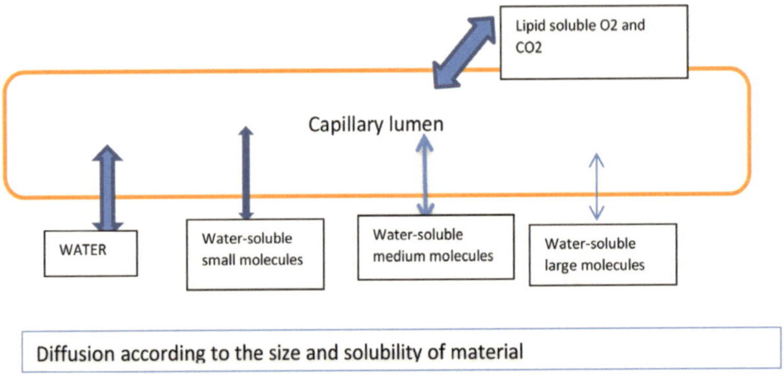

Figure 2. Diffusion according to the size and solubility of material.

The fat-soluble material does not need to pass through pores but reaches tissue directly by passing through endothelial cells. Water and water-soluble material use the pores between endothelial cells to diffuse and pass into the cell. For diffusion rate, the size of the molecule to be diffused is important (**Figure 2**).

With the Donnan effect, negatively charged proteins responsible for oncotic plasma pressure may attach to glycocalyx structures due to charge; however, they cannot bind, and plasma oncotic pressure remains high [6].

Mean values	Hydrostatic pressure	mm Hg
	Capillary	17
	Interstitial	−5.3
	Subtotal (positive = outwards)	22.3
	Osmotic pressure	
	Capillary	−28
	Interstitial	−6
	Subtotal (positive = outwards)	−22
	Total (positive = outwards)	0.3
Arterial end	Hydrostatic pressure	
	Capillary	30
	Interstitial	−5.3
	Subtotal (positive = outwards)	35.3
	Osmotic pressure	
	Capillary	−28
	Interstitial	−6
	Subtotal (positive = outwards)	−22
	Total (positive = outwards)	13.3

Venous end	Hydrostatic pressure	
	Capillary	10
	Interstitial	−5.3
	Subtotal (positive = outwards)	15.3
	Osmotic pressure	
	Capillary	−28
	Interstitial	−6
	Subtotal (positive = outwards)	−22
	Total (positive = outwards)	−6.7

Table 1. Pressure distribution in microcirculation.

Forces controlling fluid transfer in capillaries were defined by Starling. While capillary pressure (Pc) and interstitial fluid oncotic pressure (πif) ensure water and solutes leave the vein, plasma oncotic pressure (Pπ) and interstitial hydrostatic pressure (Pif) attempt to prevent water and solute transfer in the interstitial area. In conclusion, net filtration pressure (NFP) develops as NFP = Pc–Pif–π P + πif. The pressure distribution is shown in **Table 1**.

According to the Starling equation, there is 0.3 mmHg net outward pressure for 2 ml/min outward flow. The difference is removed from the interstitial area by the lymphatic system. Filtration occurs in the arteriole sections of the capillaries. Fluid reabsorption is clear at the venule tips [3].

Lymphatic capillaries include endothelial flaps, and these flaps prevent reverse leakage of fluid. Fluid flow is ensured by skeletal muscle contractions with flow rates in the interval 4–150 ml/hr. Interstitial fluid pressure and lymph fluid rate determine lymphatic flow.

2. Microcirculation regulation

In eukaryotes, transfer of oxygen and nutrition into the cell and removal of carbon dioxide and waste material occurs at the cell surface. In multicellular organisms, this event occurs in the interstitial area [3].

In humans, blood flow follows the path: left ventricle → large- and medium-diameter arteries → small arteries known as precapillary resistance arterioles and terminal arterioles → capillary beds not containing contractile elements and where oxygen and solute exchange occurs → postcapillary resistance venules and collecting veins → capacitance veins and large veins → right atrium.

Tissue oxygenation (DO2) is calculated as being equal to arterial oxygen saturation (SaO_2) × blood haemoglobin level cHb × 1.39 × cardiac output (CO).

The result is that it takes 30–60 s for oxygen entering blood in the lungs to reach tissues. However, for oxygen to reach peripheral tissues, it is necessary for there to be sufficient airway opening, normal respiratory pattern, normal alveolar gas exchange, sufficient blood haemoglobin level, and sturdy and sufficient vein structure in addition to microcirculatory blood flow supplying metabolic requirements of the tissues [7].

For metabolism and sufficient adenosine triphosphate (ATP) production to occur, tissues need to have sufficient blood perfusion. In situations without sufficient oxygen supply, anaerobic glycolysis increases in tissues and lactic acid release occurs. Increased lactic acid causes metabolic acidosis. Acidosis reduces cardiac contractility and increases peripheral vascular resistance and, as a result, tissue hypoxia deepens. At the same time, increasing blood potassium levels linked to developing acidosis reduce cardiac contractility and cause a reduction in the presentation of oxygen to tissues.

Apart from true arteriovenous shunt areas of the body, blood perfusion passes through many capillary veins, and capillary blood flow is controlled by arteriole resistance. This situation is more pronounced especially in the heart, lungs, and skeletal muscles. In situations when reduced blood flow reduces in tissues, regional vasodilatation may ensure sufficient blood perfusion of tissues and sufficient oxygenation [8].

Moving away from the arteriolar areas, smooth muscle structure begins to appear in the adventitia layer of veins. This smooth muscle structure is contracted by adrenergic stimuli and is considered to increase capillary perfusion pressure [3].

Vasoconstriction in hyperoxic situations is an attempt to keep tissue oxygenization stable and, in addition, to reduce the risk of tissue hyperoxygenization [9]. The 2.5 atmosphere pressure applied during hyperbaric oxygen treatment increases 4–5 times partial oxygen pressure in subdermal healthy and infected tissues by [10]. In a study, hyperbaric oxygen administration had reduced local blood circulation about 76.5% in pancreatitis patients, while this rate was identified as 37% with normobaric hyperoxygenization [11]. Hyperoxic situations increase oxygen amount, which dissolves in plasma. The free oxygen amount is an important point in the development of oxygen diffusion. There is a moderate level of oxygen saturation values measured in the postcapillary section of microcirculation. This effect may be explained by the vasoconstriction which occurs with the hyperbaric oxygen administration.

During inflammation increased leukocyte adhesion occurring in venules and resistance increase to venous blood flow develops and venous pressure increases. At the same time, an increase occurs in the length of venules. An attempt is made to increase oxygen presentation to tissues [12, 13]. Also during inflammation, mediators like vascular endothelial growth factor (VEGF) are released to the environment and have a venodilatatory effect.

Arterioles and terminal arterioles cause changes in local blood perfusion resistance and may directly change the blood flow amount to tissues. In situations with vasodilatation of arterioles and terminal arterioles, there is an opening of closed capillaries and lengthening of capillaries. This situation causes an increase in the surface necessary for material transfer. However, in situations with venular contraction, there is a hydrostatic pressure increase in capillary beds and diffusion pressure increases. Capacitance and large veins change cardiac output above the heart's full volume and affect microcirculation (**Figure 3**).

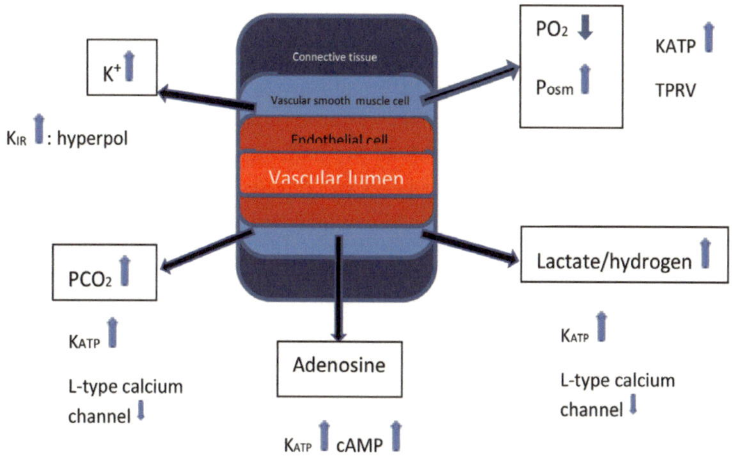

Figure 3. Local vasodilatation with tissue metabolites. K_{ATP}, ATP-dependent potassium ion channel; K_{IR}, inward-rectifying potassium ion channel that gives rise to hyperpolarization; TRPV, transitory receptor-mediated potential; cAMP, cyclic adenosine monophosphate.

As described by Bayliss, in situations with increased blood pressure, an attempt is made to keep blood flow to vital organs like the brain, heart, kidneys, liver, and carotid bodies fixed via developing vasocontraction [14]. This adaptation is processed in reverse in hypotensive situations. In this development, the tension-sensitive sodium and calcium channels play a role.

2.1. Factors affecting arteriole resistance

- Autonomous nervous system (cholinergic, adrenergic, non-cholinergic, non-adrenergic system)
- Vasoactive humoral and tissue factors (angiotensin II, bradykinin, vasopressin, catecholamines, natriuretic peptides, etc.)
- Local metabolic changes (partial oxygen pressure [PO2], partial carbon dioxide pressure [PCO2], pH, osmotic pressure [Posm], potassium [K+] concentration, metabolic material like adenosine)

In endothelial tissue, the friction caused by blood triggers nitric oxide (NO) release. In situations with vasodilatation in NO terminal arterioles, increasing NO release develops. Friction-linked vasodilatation is responsible for mechanoconduction of the glycocalyx structure covering the endothelial surface and plays a role in blood flow regulation in inflammation, ischemia and other pathological situations [15].

Vasodilators like NO and prostaglandin I2 are found in the whole vascular system, especially the terminal arterioles. Other vasodilator effect agonists include serotonin, histamine, adenosine triphosphate (ATP), adenosine diphosphate (ADP), bradykinin, acetylcholine, thrombin, and endothelin.

NO formed by the nitric oxide synthase enzyme found within endothelial cells is effective through paracrine routes. NO within the cell commonly shows the effect by ensuring calcium entry into the cell via guanosine monophosphate and protein kinase activation. In addition to vasodilatation, NO has anti-thrombogenic effects by reducing tissue factor expression, platelet aggregation, and adhesion molecule expression like VCAM. At the same time, proliferation in venous smooth muscles is reduced and it limits neointimal hyperplasia development in vein walls [16].

As a result of material like adrenalin, thrombin, and angiotensin II binding to receptors found in abluminal vascular smooth muscle cells, calcium entry into the cell is activated and due to the inositol triphosphate (IP3) pathway, endothelin released into the subendothelial interstitial areas causes the better-known vasoconstriction effect [17]. In situations where vasodilator materials pass through endothelial cells with increased permeability outside of the vein, the vasodilator effect reverses and may cause vasoconstriction.

Specific receptor expression available in endothelial and smooth muscle tissue found in the vein structures of organs affect agonist concentration and provide vasoactive material to luminal and abluminal vein structures affecting the concentration or dilatation response [3].

In 1922, August Krogh et al. first defined vasodilatation occurring due to the chemical stimulus. In 1971, Siggins and Weitsen showed that vasodilatation was caused by cholinergic stimulation. Khayutin et al. in 1991 showed that vasodilatation occurred due to myelin nerve stimulus. In 1959, Hilton showed that communication present between the smooth muscle cells found in the vascular walls was effective on vasodilatation.

Gap junctions are structures formed by two half channels completing each other with nearly 9 nm size, allowing transfer between cells of ions and molecules with weight lower than 1 kDa isolated from the extracellular environment and linking two neighbouring cells. Just as gap junctions form between the same type of cells (endothelium-endothelium, smooth muscle-smooth muscle, etc.), they may also form between different cells (myoendothelial gap junctions). The channels allow transfer between cells of electrical stimuli and calcium [18].

Each half of gap junctions found in vein structures contain six connexins (Cx) proteins (Cx39, Cx40, Cx43, Cx45) [19]. Each connexin protein has effects with different clinical results [20].

In development-linked vasodilatation, each agonist has a different effect mechanism, with the best-described effect mechanism belonging to the agonist acetylcholine. When acetylcholine binds to a G protein-dependent muscarinic receptor, inositol triphosphate phosphorylation develops causing calcium release from endothelial endoplasmic reticulum [21, 22]. Simultaneously, calcium-dependent potassium channels open leading to hyperpolarization development in the cell [23]. After this flow, vasodilatation develops causing closure of voltage-dependent calcium channels within endothelial and vein smooth muscle cells [24]. At the same time, ion flows are communicated between cells via gap junctions with vasodilatation spreading distal and proximal to the point of acetylcholine binding [2].

Pericytes found in venules have regulatory effects on proliferation, differentiation and contractility of endothelial cells. During new vein creation, in situations where the endothelial layer is developing with tube shape contacts pericytes, endothelial growth and proliferation are suppressed, and maturation of the endothelial basal membrane structure is ensured [25, 26].

In situations with low oxygen levels or pH, ATP molecules released from erythrocytes found in microcirculation cause vasodilatation while haemoglobin molecules occurring with erythrocyte fragmentation bind to NO causing the development of NO-dependent vasodilatation.

During hyperoxia the reactive oxygen radicals prevent nitric oxide-mediated vasodilatation; on the other hand, vascoconstrictor effect results in low tissue blood flow [27]. In addition, synthesis of the vasodilator prostaglandin is reduced while synthesis of the vasoconstrictor prostaglandin (and endothelin-1) is increased [28].

3. Methods to assess microcirculation flow

The microcirculation performs the necessary oxygen distribution to meet the basic metabolic requirements of the tissues. Anatomically, it consists of arterioles, capillaries and venules. In situations where physiological or pathological stress develops, the balance between oxygen delivery and demand becomes very important. This delicate balance can play an important role in the progression of critical illnesses. In daily clinical practice, monitoring the microcirculation is essential for detection of potential organ dysfunctions. The ideal technique would allow quantification of vascular recruitment and the magnitude, heterogeneity, responsiveness, and efficiency of oxygen transfer to the tissues. There are a variety of methods and parameters available to evaluate the microcirculatory state of a patient.

4. Assessment of microcirculation

The assessment of these factors can be analysed in five parameters: (i) total microvascular density (TVD), (ii) perfused microvascular density (PVD), (iii) proportion of perfused microvessels (PPV), (iv) microvascular flow index (MFI) and (v) heterogeneity of microvascular flow index. The first two reflect density, (iii) and (iv) reflect the flow, and (v) represents the heterogeneity of flow. Microcirculatory blood flow can be detected at the bedside by videomicroscopic techniques, and by laser Doppler flowmetry, near-infrared spectroscopy (NIRS), tissue reflectance spectrophotometry, or by tonometry. These techniques provide simple and quantitative data. Biochemical parameters that show microcirculation are reliable and include lactate, tissue CO_2 content and venous oxygen saturation.

5. Direct methods

5.1. Measuring microcirculatory perfusion

Video microscopic techniques involve highly sensitive video microscopes that allow direct measurement of capillary density, perfusion and flow dynamics. Video microscopic techniques have shown a correlation between increased mortality in ICU patients [29]. These techniques, which included orthogonal polarisation spectral (OPS), sidestream dark-field (SDF) imaging and incident dark-field (IDF) imaging (CytoCam) provide in vivo visualisation of the microcirculation. OPS and SDF imaging have become clinically useless due to the large size, motion and pressure artefacts, operator-dependent output, and the need for offline analysis, which takes time to produce data.

6. Indirect methods

6.1. Measuring elements of tissue oxygenation

There are quite some methodologies available for estimating or measuring tissue oxygenation at the different levels.

Central venous oxygen saturation ($ScvO_2$) and mixed venous oxygen saturation (SvO_2).

They provide knowledge of the patient's oxygen delivery, oxygen consumption, and cardiac output. $ScvO_2 > 70\%$ or $SvO_2 > 65\%$ is recommended for critical patients [30]. SvO_2 is an adaptive variable depending on four elementary-regulated components: the real O_2 consumption, SaO_2, haemoglobin and cardiac output. Consequently, SvO_2 (or its surrogate $ScvO_2$) is widely fluctuating. Thus, when normal, those parameters cannot rule out any impairment in tissue oxygenation related to an impaired microcirculation [31].

6.2. Near-infrared spectroscopy (NIRS)

NIRS has been developed as a non-invasive diagnostic tool for measurement of regional haemoglobin oxygen saturation in a particular organ. NIRS is mainly used in the evaluation of cerebral oxygenation in cardiac, non-cardiac surgery and traumatic intensive care patients. The NIRS signal is restricted to vessels that have a diameter of less than 1 mm, and this technique is not suitable for states of heterogeneous blood flow [32]. Tissue O_2 saturation (StO_2) mostly describes the saturation of all vessels, while total tissue haemoglobin (HbT) and the tissue haemoglobin index (THI) indicate the amount of blood present in the tested region. Brain venous blood is primarily responsible for a decrease in brain saturation and predominantly results from a local increase in oxygen extraction. During haemorrhage the arterial component preserved while venous part decreases markedly. On the other hand, in trauma patients, StO_2 is altered only in the severe cases and in other forms show low sensitivity [33]. NIRS-derived dynamic measurements (vaso-occlusive test, VOT) demonstrated profound alterations in microvascular reactivity. The NIRS technique is done for a brief episode of forearm ischemia induced by transient inflation of a cuff determines changes in StO_2. Some indices can be measured during this test, but the most important is the ascending slope reflecting microvascular reactivity. The severity of these alterations in microvascular reactivity is associated with organ dysfunction and mortality [34].

6.3. Tissue CO_2 (gastric tonometry, veno-arterial CO_2 gradient, transcutaneous CO_2)

Tissue PCO_2 ($PtCO_2$) has been measured in the stomach, sublingual area, and earlobe. Tissue PCO_2 has three major elements: VCO_2, $PaCO_2$, and tissue blood flow. Normally, an increase

http://dx.doi.org/10.5772/intechopen.75609

in tissue metabolism (VCO2) increases tissue perfusion and decreases PCO_2. When $PaCO_2$ is constant, and $PtCO_2$ is increased, there is an inadequate relationship between metabolism and tissue perfusion. Normal tissue-arterial CO_2 gradient (PCO_2 gap) <7 mmHg. Elevated PCO_2 gaps may signify either flow stagnation or tissue hypoxia [35]. Importantly, there is an inverse relationship between microvascular perfusion and the PCO_2 gap. $PtCO_2$ consequently represents a good assessment of tissue perfusion.

Microcirculatory alterations in critically ill patients may play a role in the development of organ dysfunction. Video microscopic techniques and tissue PCO2 measurements can be used to evaluate microvascular perfusion. But, microcirculation monitoring is not yet part of routine clinical practice.

6.4. Lactate

Lactate in the human body is a metabolic product of anaerobic glycolysis, produced from the reduction of pyruvate by the enzyme lactate dehydrogenase, and reflects inadequate oxygen delivery. Normally, a total amount of 1500 mmol of lactate is produced daily in adult, and blood lactate levels are sustained less than 2 mmol/L. However, in the state of hypoperfusion and hypoxia, pyruvate rapidly accumulate, and its metabolism is shifted almost entirely to lactate production. The tissue hypoxia is a cause of lactate elevation and characterised by supply-dependent oxygen consumption [36]. Single measurement of lactate can only serve as a risk-stratification biomarker. Lactate clearance with its association with clinical outcome should be used during treatment to make it more clinically useful [37].

6.5. Microcirculation and hyperbaric oxygen therapy

Hyperbaric oxygen therapy (HBOT) is a clinical treatment in which a patient breathes pure oxygen for a limited period of time at an increased pressure. This therapy has been suggested to improve oxygen supply to tissues and therefore improves microcirculation [38]. HBOT in patients with diabetic foot ulcer was associated with a greater reduction in the ulcer wound area than standard therapy and significantly improves the ulcers in a short term [39]. Also, HBOT which is applied in acute ischemic stroke, femoral head necrosis, and carbon monoxide intoxication aims to increase oxygen supply to the ischemic tissue and to reduce the extent of irreversible tissue damage [40–42].

7. Microcirculation and disease

7.1. Microcirculatory dysfunction

Microcirculation plays a critical role in the physiological process such as oxygen supply to tissues and nutritional exchange and has a key role in modulation of inflammation and coagulation. These functions are mainly controlled by endothelial cells, which produce biologic signals to regulate local blood flow, cell adhesion, permeability, and coagulation activation. The most important function of the microcirculation is the regulation of flow within the different organs [43].

Microcirculation, in general, provides sufficient oxygen distribution to meet the oxygen demands of every cell within an organ. A regulatory mechanism with several signalling pathways allows microcirculatory flow to occur independently of changes in systemic blood pressure; this mechanism is called autoregulation. Perfusion of capillaries increases due to the vasodilation of terminal arterioles, which causes a decrease in the number of recruited capillaries. These capillaries are mainly under local control, which is possible because endothelial cells sense metabolic and physical signals, and respond to them by modulating arteriolar smooth muscle cell tone. In this process, nitric oxide (NO), which is produced by endothelial cells, is one of the components in the exertion of this process [44].

In the pathophysiology of sepsis and septic shock, the microcirculation is the basic region of the circulatory system, in which main components are arterioles, venules, shunts, and capillaries. The structures in the microcirculation system are capable of contraction, except capillaries. Capillaries are made of endothelial cells alone, without contractile structures. Microcirculatory dysfunction may arise as a result of several factors such as endothelial dysfunction, leukocyte-endothelium interactions, coagulation and inflammatory disorders, and functional shunting that may occur during sepsis which can affect capillaries to change hemodynamics [43, 44].

Microcirculatory changes during sepsis include various mechanisms such as redistribution of blood flow from the skin and the splanchnic area to brain or heart, or with endothelial activation and injury which results with the loss of the glycocalyx around endothelium. Increased microvascular permeability with capillary damage then causes oedema formation and hypovolemia. And also, secondary capillary plugging comes out with decreased RBC deformability and increased leukocyte adhesion to the endothelial surface. On the other hand, production of reactive oxygen species (ROS) disturbs microcirculatory structures, cellular interactions, and haemostasis. Overall, these alterations contribute to a reduction in decreased functional capillary density, the progress of various abnormalities in microcirculatory blood flow, and the loss of main vasoregulation in most vascular beds. These alterations terminate with a disrupted regulation of local oxygen delivery, which turns into the fast initiation of tissue hypoxia [44, 47].

Proinflammatory cytokines become dominant in the early stages of sepsis to eliminate the pathogen. However, proinflammatory responses in sepsis generate an intense response that impairs the microcirculation. In this stage, most of the cellular components of the microcirculation, such as endothelial cells, smooth muscle cells, platelets, leukocytes, and red blood cells are affected. Increased number of interrupted capillaries results with microcirculatory dysfunction which appears to have prognostic significance in sepsis, as the severity of initial microcirculatory imbalance in the early resuscitation phase of therapy [45, 46].

In sepsis, NO synthase (iNOS) which heterogeneously expressed in various vascular beds, causes pathological shunts. Therefore, iNOS-deficient areas become hypoperfused. Furthermore, increased production of reactive oxygen species interferes with NO formation by endothelial NOS and with formed NO, reducing its concentration. Also, during sepsis, red blood cells lose their ability to release vasodilators in the presence of hypoxia that impairs physiological regulatory mechanism of microcirculation. In that case, red blood cells become less deformable and more easily aggregate with endothelial cells during sepsis [47, 49].

During sepsis, the percentage of activated neutrophils with increased adhesion molecules generate reactive oxygen species and inflammatory soluble factors that directly disrupt microcirculatory structures, such as the endothelial glycocalyx. Oxidative stress causes changes in endothelial glycocalyx structure. Permanent glycocalyx degradation leads to loss of integrity of adherens junctions and increased paracellular permeability with the following break of endothelial barrier function, which results in fluid leakage from the intravascular space and causes tissue oedema. Afterwards, accumulation of water in tissues leads to tissue hypoxia.

In sepsis, endothelial glycocalyx degradation is associated with sepsis-related clinical conditions such as acute lung injury and cardiovascular dysfunction as a consequence of microcirculation dysfunction. Also, glycocalyx degradation contributes to the enhanced expression of adhesion molecules with increased leukocyte trafficking and shift towards the procoagulant state. Prothrombotic effect further contributes the adhesion of red blood cells, leukocytes, and platelets to the vascular endothelium, which causes vascular microthrombosis. The activation of coagulation pathways results in capillary obstruction by fibrin clots secondary to disseminated intravascular coagulation [44, 47].

7.2. Treatment

The microcirculation is important for the normal delivery of oxygen to vital organs. The type and phase of critical illness define the degree of microcirculatory resuscitation required. It is important to recruit the microcirculation due to heterogeneous nature of the microvascular alterations. Fluid resuscitation and vasoactive agents are one of the main therapies for the hemodynamic resuscitation that aims to restore the circulating volume, and increasing the cardiac output and arterial blood pressure in shock patients and play a critical role with the goal of improving tissue perfusion. Individual responses to vasopressors may change, but the microvascular response to vasopressors appears to be dependent on the basal condition of the microcirculation [50]. Fluid resuscitation improves microcirculatory blood flow. The mechanisms by which fluids may improve the microcirculation are not well understood but may be related to restoring circulatory volume which increases perfusion pressure and causes local vasodilation, or modulates interactions between the endothelium and circulating cells to decrease microvascular blood viscosity [46, 48, 49].

Hypertonic saline (HTS) is a potential solution to cure the microcirculation of traumatic haemorrhagic shock. HTS improves intestinal perfusion associated with arteriolar vasodilation of distal premucosal arterioles, decreases endothelial oedema and prevents leukocyte adhesion to postcapillary venules. To restore capillary density, a new approach to fluid resuscitation is based on the fluid with high viscosity to increase plasma viscosity and NO production causing microcirculatory vasodilation with resulting capillary recruitment. At the same time, vasopressor agents may maintain tissue perfusion in the presence of life-threatening hypotension in haemorrhagic shock, even if fluid dilatation is in progress and hypovolemia has not yet been corrected [49].

The effects of red blood cell transfusions also seem to be quite variable. One of the other commonly used therapy is transfusions of red blood cells (RBC), which is used in critically ill patients to restore oxygen-carrying capacity. But, transfusion decisions are based on serum haemoglobin levels, and it is difficult to notice because normal microvascular haematocrit is much lower than systemic values. Although the beneficial effect of RBC transfusions over microcirculatory parameters in septic patients is still not clear, RBC transfusions are effective in improving tissue oxygen transport by promoting RBC delivery to the microcirculation [50].

Fluid resuscitation in combination with vasoactive and inotropic support is effective in improving the microcirculation. Recruitment of the microcirculation can be achieved with combination therapies. An anti-inflammatory agent or specific iNOS inhibitor can reduce pathological shunting and improve blood flow to recruit weak microcirculatory units. The effects can be seen in the early phase of sepsis, within 24 h of diagnosis, but if cardiac output is increased, no improvement will be made after 48 h [51].

The use of steroids in sepsis may provide a clinical benefit in modulating the systemic inflammatory response. It can preserve the endothelial glycocalyx and attenuate rolling of leucocytes to the endothelium, may improve endothelial function and thereby ameliorate the distributive defect [52].

Statins, which are cholesterol-lowering agents also have pleiotropic effects and have an anti-inflammatory and anti-oxidant activity during sepsis. They increase levels of eNOS, with the down-regulation of iNOS, so this regulation of NOS increases NO levels, restoring the autoregulatory functions [53].

Vasodilator substances may have a role to restore the microcirculation and decrease the effect of excessive vasoconstriction which causes decreased vascular density and stopped-flow capillaries. In a research, it was reported that nitroglycerin administration rapidly improved the microcirculation [54].

In haemorrhagic shock, reducing the blood flow to the microvascular units may prevent hypoxia. This downregulation of cellular metabolism is called conformance or hibernation. However, increase in lactate level during the acute phase of haemorrhagic shock indicates the limits of this adaptative metabolic downregulation. The critical factor in microvascular regulation to meet oxygen supply is the local regulation of arteriolar tone. Many mechanisms contribute to the local regulation of arteriolar tone, which includes response to myogenic response, shear-dependent response, and tissue metabolic response. During haemorrhagic shock, the decrease in DO2 reduces the generation of adenosine 5′ triphosphate (ATP) and adenosine 5′ diphosphate (ADP) which results in the accumulation of ADP and its degradation products. CO_2 is a strong vasodilator, which accumulates when there is an increase in cellular metabolism or reduced clearance of CO_2 during tissue hypoperfusion. In haemorrhagic shock, the therapeutic precedence is to stop the bleeding and to prevent the increase of bleeding. Fluid resuscitation may promote coagulopathy by diluting coagulation factors [55, 56].

Reduced microvascular perfusion is a characteristic feature of sepsis and implicated in organ dysfunction with multiple organ failure. Hyperbaric oxygen (HBO) has potentially beneficial effects for the microcirculation improvement in sepsis . It was shown that HBOT improves microcirculation independently from systemic hemodynamic parameters which is a key therapeutic target in septic shock patients. [57]. Some of well-documented HBOT mechanisms in sepsis treatment are attenuation of inflammatory mediators and free radicals, reduction of bacterial proliferation, inhibition of lipopolysaccharide-induced acute lung injury and enabling neutrophils to kill bacteria with oxygen dependent mechanisms. It was also proposed that HBOT can delay onset of sepsis and may boost the effect of antibiotics [58].

Meningococcal sepsis can cause purpura fulminans which occurs by the formation of thrombi haemorrhages and occlusion of dermal vessels and often a life-threatening condition [59].. Clinically, it was shown that HBOT is effective in meningococcal sepsis which is complicated with the necrotic tissue [60]. HBOT with its immunostimulatory, neovascularity, and bactericidal effect can be adjunct treatment for non-healing ulcers and problematic wounds.

8. Conclusion

In conclusion, microcirculation plays a critical role in the physiological process such as oxygen supply to vital organs, nutritional exchange and modulation of inflammation. The most important function of the microcirculation is the regulation of flow within the different organs. Microcirculatory changes include various mechanisms such as redistribution of blood flow from the skin and the splanchnic area to brain or heart, or with endothelial activation and injury which results with the loss of the glycocalyx around endothelium. The assessment of the microcirculation enables us for the early detection of possible deterioration and potential organ dysfunctions. Microcirculatory blood flow can be detected at the bedside by different techniques which are simple and gives quantitative data. Fluid resuscitation and vasoactive agents are one of the main therapies for the hemodynamic resuscitation that aims to restore the circulating volume, and increasing the cardiac output and arterial blood pressure and play a critical role with the goal of improving tissue perfusion. HBOT inhibits replicating, spreading of anaerobic and some other bacteria and is a clinical treatment adjunct to traditional surgery and antibiotic therapy for the deadly serious necrotizing infection. Also, HBOT applied in acute ischemic stroke, femoral head necrosis and carbon monoxide intoxication aim to increase oxygen supply to the ischemic tissue and to reduce the extent of irreversible tissue damage.

Author details

Fethi Gul[1]*, Omer Faruk Boran[2] and Reyhan Arslantas[3]

*Address all correspondence to: gulfethi@gmail.com

1 Marmara University, Department of Anesthesiology and Reanimation, Istanbul, Turkey

2 Sutcu Imam University, Department of Anestehesiology and Reanimation, Kahramanmaras, Turkey

3 Health Sciences University, Kartal Dr. Lutfi Kırdar Training and Research Hospital, Anesthesiology and Reanimation Clinics, Istanbul, Turkey

References

[1] Guyton and Hall Textbook of Medical Physiology 11th Edition: section 16

[2] Steven S. Regulation of blood flow in the microcirculation. Microcirculation. 2005;**12**:33-45

[3] Jacob et al. Regulation of blood flow and volume exchange across the microcirculation. Critical Care. 2016;**20**:319

[4] Scallan J, Huxley VH, Korthuis RJ. Capillary Fluid Exchange: Regulation, Functions, and Pathology. Morgan & Claypool Life Sciences. 1st Edition: Section 1.2. 2010

[5] Gill AL, Bell CNA. Hyperbaric oxygen: Its uses, mechanisms of action and outcomes. QJM: An International Journal of Medicine. 2004;**97**(7):385-395

[6] RM B, Koeppen BM, Stanton BA. Physiology. 4th ed. Vol. 1998. pp. 217-221

[7] Chawla LS, Ince C, Chappell D, Gan TJ, Kellum JA, Mythen M. Vascular content, tone, integrity, and haemodynamics for guiding fluid therapy: A conceptual approach. British Journal of Anaesthesia. 2014;**113**:748-755

[8] Secomb TW. Theoretical models for regulation of blood flow. Microcirculation. 2008; **15**:765-775

[9] Stirban A, Lentrod S. Functional changes in microcirculation during hyperbaric and normobaric oxygen therapy. Undersea and Hyperbaric Medikal Society. 2009;**36**:5-9

[10] Korhonen K, Kuttila K, Niinikoski J. Tissue gas tensions in patients with necrotising fasciitis and healthy controls during treatment with hyperbaric oxygen: A clinical study. The European Journal of Surgery. 2000;**166**:530-534

[11] Cuthbertson CM, Su KH, Muralidharan V, Millar I, Malcontenti-Wilson C, Christophi C. Hyperbaric oxygen improves capillary morphology in severe acute pancreatitis. Pancreas. 2008;**36**:70-75

[12] Habazettl H, Kupatt C, Zahler S, Becker BF, Messmer K. Selectins and beta 2-integrins mediate post-ischaemic venular adhesion of polymorphonuclear leukocytes, but not capillary plugging, in isolated hearts. Pflügers Archiv. 1999;**438**:479-485

[13] Ezaki T, Baluk P, Thurston G, La Barbara A, Woo C, McDonald DM. Time course of endothelial cell proliferation and microvascular remodeling in chronic inflammation. The American Journal of Pathology. 2001;**158**:2043-2055

[14] Bayliss WM. On the local reactions of the arterial wall to changes of internal pressure. The Journal of Physiology. 1902;**28**(3):220-231

[15] Becker BF, Chappell D, Jacob M. Endothelial glycocalyx and coronary vascular permeability: The fringe benefit. Basic Research in Cardiology. 2010;**105**:687-701

[16] Somani A et al. The dynamic regulation of microcirculatory conduit function:Features relevant to transfusion medicine. Transfusion and Apheresis Science. 2010;**431**:61-68

[17] Davenport AP, Hyndman KA, Dhaun N, Southan C, Kohan DE, Pollock JS, et al. Endothelin. Pharmacological Reviews. 2016;**68**:357-418

[18] Bagher P, Segal SS. Regulation of blood flow in the microcirculation: Role of conducted vasodilation. Acta Physiologica. 2011;**202**:271-284

[19] Little TL, Beyer EC, Duling BR. Connexin 43 and connexin 40 gap junctional proteins are present in arteriolar smooth muscle and endothelium in vivo. The American Journal of Physiology. 1995a;**268**:729-739

[20] Figueroa XFDBR. Dissection of two Cx37- independent conducted vasodilator mechanisms by deletion of Cx40: Electrotonic versus regenerative conduction. American Journal of Physiology. Heart and Circulatory Physiology. 2008;**295**:2001-2007

[21] Danthuluri NR, Cybulsky MI, Brock TA. Achinduced calcium transients in primary cultures of rabbit aortic endothelial cells. American Journal of Physiology. Heart and Circulatory Physiology. 1988;**255**:1549-1553

[22] Himmel HM, Whorton AR, Strauss HC. Intracellular calcium, currents, and stimulus-response coupling in endothelial cells. Hypertension. 1993;**21**:112-127

[23] Busse R, Fichtner H, Luckhoff A, Kohlhardt M. Hyperpolarization and increased free calcium in acetylcholine- stimulated endothelial cells. American Journal of Physiology. Heart and Circulatory Physiology. 1988;**255**:965-969

[24] Ledoux J, Werner ME, Brayden JE, Nelson MT. Calcium-activated potassium channels and the regulation of vascular tone. Physiology. 2006;**21**:69-78

[25] Orlidge A, D'Amore PA. Inhibition of capillary endothelial cell growth by pericytes and smooth muscle cells. The Journal of Cell Biology. 1987;**105**:1455-1462

[26] Sato Y, Rifkin DB. Inhibition of endothelial cell movement by pericytes and smooth muscle cells: Activation of a latent transforming growth factor-beta 1-like molecule by plasmin during co-culture. The Journal of Cell Biology. 1989;**109**:309-315

[27] Katusic ZS, Vanhoutte PM. Superoxide anion is an endothelium-derived contracting factor. The American Journal of Physiology. 1989;**257**:33-37

[28] Lund V, Kentala E, Scheinin H, Klossner J, Koskinen P, Jalonen J. Effect of hyperbaric conditions on plasma stress hormone levels and endothelin-1. Undersea & Hyperbaric Medicine. 1999;**26**:87-92

[29] Vellinga NA, Boerma EC, Koopmans M, et al. International study on microcirculatory shock occurrence in acutely ill patients. Critical Care Medicine. 2015;**43**:48-56

[30] Squara P. Central venous oxygenation: When physiology explains apparent discrepancies. Critical Care. 2014;**18**(6):579

[31] Pope JV, Jones AE, Gaieski DF, et al. Multicenter study of central venous oxygen saturation [ScvO[2]] as a predictor of mortality in patients with sepsis. Annals of Emergency Medicine. 2010;**55**:40-46

[32] De Backer D, Ospina-Tascon G, Salgado D, Favory R, Creteur J, Vincent JL. Monitoring the microcirculation in the critically ill patient: Current methods and future approaches. Intensive Care Medicine 2010;**36**:1813-1182

[33] Crookes BA, Cohn SM, Bloch S, et al. Can near-infrared spectroscopy identify the severity of shock in trauma patients? The Journal of Trauma. 2005;**58**:806-813

[34] Creteur J, Carollo T, Soldati G, et al. The prognostic value of muscle StO[2] in septic patients. Intensive Care Medicine. 2007;**33**:1549-1556

[35] Schlichtig R, Bowles SA. Distinguishing between aerobic and anaerobic appearance of dissolved CO2 in intestine during low flow. Journal of Applied Physiology. 1994;**76**:2443e51

[36] Cain SM. Oxygen delivery and uptake in dogs during anemic and hypoxic hypoxia. Journal of Applied Physiology: Respiratory, Environmental and Exercise Physiology. 1977;**42**:228-234

[37] Slottosch I, Liakopoulos O, Kuhn E, Scherner M, Deppe AC, Sabashnikov A, et al. Lactate and lactate clearance as valuable tool to evaluate ECMO therapy in cardiogenic shock. Journal of Critical Care. 2017;**42**:35-41

[38] Milstein DM, Helmers R, Hackmann S, Belterman CN, van Hulst RA, de Lange J. Sublingual microvascular perfusion is altered during normobaric and hyperbaric hyperoxia. Microvascular Research. 2016;**105**:93-102

[39] Kranke P, Bennett MH, Martyn-St James M, Schnabel A, Debus SE, Weibel S. Hyperbaric oxygen therapy for chronic wounds. Cochrane Database of Systematic Reviews. 2015;**24**(6):5-6

[40] Poli S, Veltkamp R. Oxygen therapy in acute ischemic stroke – Experimental efficacy and molecular mechanisms. Current Molecular Medicine. 2009;**9**(2):227-241

[41] Li W, Ye Z, Wang W, Wang K, Li L, Zhao D. Clinical effect of hyperbaric oxygen therapy in the treatment of femoral head necrosis : A systematic review and meta-analysis. Der Orthopäde. 2017;**46**(5):440-446

[42] Bleecker ML. Carbon monoxide intoxication. Handbook of Clinical Neurology. 2015; **131**:191-203

[43] De Backer D, Donadello K, Sakr Y, Ospina-Tascon G, Salgado D, Scolletta S, Vincent JL. Microcirculatory alterations in patients with severe sepsis: Impact of time of assessment and relationship with outcome. Critical Care Medicine. 2013;**41**:791-799

[44] Bateman RM, Jagger JE, Sharpe MD, Ellsworth ML, Mehta S, Ellis CG. Erythrocyte deformability is a nitric oxide-mediated factor in decreased capillary density during sepsis. American Journal of Physiology. Heart and Circulatory Physiology. 2001;**280**:2848-2856

[45] Borutaite V, Matthias A, Harris H, Moncada S, Brown GC. Reversible inhibition of cellular respiration by nitric oxide in vascular inflammation. American Journal of Physiology. Heart and Circulatory Physiology. 2001;**281**:2256-2260

[46] Constantinescu AA, Vink H, Spaan JA. Endothelial cell glycocalyx modulates immobilization of leukocytes at the endothelial surface. Arteriosclerosis, Thrombosis, and Vascular Biology. 2003;**23**:1541-1547

[47] Cabrales P, Vázquez BY, Tsai AG, Intaglietta M. Microvascular and capillary perfusion following glycocalyx degradation. Journal of Applied Physiology. 2007;**102**:2251-2259

[48] Cepinskas G, Wilson JX. Inflammatory response in microvascular endothelium in sepsis: Role of oxidants. Journal of Clinical Biochemistry and Nutrition. 2008;**42**:175-184

[49] Doerschug KC, Delsing AS, Schmidt GA, Haynes WG. Impairments in microvascular reactivity are related to organ failure in human sepsis. American Journal of Physiology. Heart and Circulatory Physiology. 2007;**293**:1065-1071

[50] Kanoore Edul VS, Dubin A, Ince C. The microcirculation as a therapeutic target in the treatment of sepsis and shock. Seminars in Respiratory and Critical Care Medicine. 2011;**32**:558-568

[51] Dubin A, Pozo MO, Casabella CA, Murias G, Pálizas F, Moseinco MC, Kanoore Edul VS, Estenssoro E, Ince C. Comparison of 6% hydroxyethyl starch 130/04 and saline solution for resuscitation of the microcirculation during the early goal-directed therapy of septic patients. Journal of Critical Care. 2010;**25**:659

[52] Trzeciak S, Cinel I, Phillip Dellinger R, Shapiro NI, Arnold RC, Parrillo JE, Hollenberg SM. Resuscitating the microcirculation in sepsis: The central role of nitric oxide, emerging concepts for novel therapies, and challenges for clinical trials. Academic Emergency Medicine. 2008;**15**(5):399-413

[53] Bhagat K, Vallance P. Inflammatory cytokines impair endothelium- dependent dilatation in human veins in vivo. Circulation. 1997;**96**:3042-3047

[54] Boerma EC, Ince C. The role of vasoactive agents in the resuscitation of microvascular perfusion and tissue oxygenation in critically ill patients. Intensive Care Medicine. 2010;**36**:2004-2018

[55] Boerma EC, Koopmans M, Konijn A, Kaiferova K, Bakker AJ, Van Roon EN, Buter H, Bruins N, Egbers PH, Gerritsen RT, et al. Effects of nitroglycerin on sublingual microcirculatory blood flow in patients with severe sepsis/ septic shock after a strict resuscitation protocol: A double-blind randomized placebo controlled trial. Critical Care Medicine. 2010;**38**:93-100

[56] Trzeciak S, Dellinger RP, Parrillo JE, Guglielmi M, Bajaj J, Abate NL, Arnold RC, Colilla S, Zanotti S, Hollenberg SM. Early microcirculatory perfusion derangements in patients with severe sepsis and septic shock: Relationship to hemodynamics, oxygen transport, and survival. Annals of Emergency Medicine. 2007;**49**:88-98

[57] Ferré F, Silva S, Ruiz J, Mari A, Mathe O, Sanchez-Verlaan P, Riu-Poulenc B, Fourcade O. Microcirculatory effect of hyperbaric oxygen therapy in septic patients. Critical Care. 2011;**15**(Suppl 1):284

[58] Igor A, Michael S, Stuart M, Chi T, George H. New roles of Hyperbarıc oxygen in Sepsıs. Chest. 2007;**132**(4):557

[59] Mathieu C, Olivier JL, Herve Le′ cuyer, Sandrine B, Stefano M, Xavier N. Pathogenesis of Meningococcemia. Cold Spring Harbor Perspectives in Medicine .2013;3:012393

[60] Alex PB, Tom B, Banwarı A. Purpura Fulminans in Sepsis. The American Journal of the Medical Sciences. 2006;**332**(6):339-345

Chapter 5

Cell Culture Effects of Altered Oxygen Levels and Hyperbaric Treatment *In Vitro*

Edit Gara

Additional information is available at the end of the chapter

http://dx.doi.org/10.5772/intechopen.75378

Abstract

Hyperbaric oxygen therapy (HBOT) is a state-of-the-art medical treatment, which is proved to be beneficial in a number of diseases and promising in new fields as well. HBOT is evidence-based treatment for, among others, severe CO intoxication, decompression disease and chronic wound healing. Recent studies promise beneficial effects of HBOT in multiple sclerosis. *In vitro*, cellular models of these complex pathological conditions are limited. In this chapter, we aim to mirror *in vitro* effects of HBOT and other altered oxygen levels on endothelial cells, fibroblast, mesenchymal and pluripotent stem cells. Through these *in vitro* models, the role of HBOT in angiogenesis, blot clotting, wound healing, cell therapy and tissue engineering will be discussed. To summarize *in vitro* effects of HBOT, it has beneficial role on proliferation and viability of most cell types. Furthermore, functional characteristics of the investigated cell types, for example, angiogenesis by endothelial cells, are improved in response to HBOT. Standardized preclinical protocols with HBOT help to translate the benefits to clinical trials and clinical use.

Keywords: hyperbaric oxygen, normoxia, hypoxia, *in vitro*, endothelial cells, fibroblasts, mesenchymal stem cells, endothelial differentiation, wound healing, angiogenesis

1. Introduction

Hyperbaric oxygen therapy (HBOT) is a state-of-the-art medical treatment, which has advantageous therapeutic effects in wide range of pathologies. Despite its high therapeutic potential, its availability is still restricted, and the use of hyperbaric oxygen requires significant organizing steps in most health care systems. Thus, emergent or urgent utilization is very limited.

HBOT may be used by pulmonologists, internal medicine specialists, surgeons and obstetrics as well. Evidence-based medicine recommends its use in decompression sickness to protect severe lung injury and to enhance recompression [1]. Carbon monoxide intoxication is another severe, life-threatening emergency scenario, where HBOT enhances CO discard and saves lives [2]. HBOT is recommended in severe carbon monoxide intoxication when conservative ventilation techniques are not efficient to eliminate CO, linked with hemoglobin. These time-sensitive conditions shout for widely available HBOT; however, in low-income countries, its use is still optional.

Interestingly, HBOT proved to be effective in wound healing applications, for example, ulcers, scar formation after burn injury or plastic surgery operations [3]. Cardiovascular diseases are the leading cause of death in industrialized countries. Peripheral atherosclerotic diseases and diabetes often go side-by-side. Additionally, venous circulation may also be impaired in these patients. Considering the high burden of cardiovascular diseases, number of patients suffering from not-healing ulcers is constantly increasing. Furthermore, retinal arterial stenosis severely impairs vision, in which condition HBOT is on the palette of treatment applications. Wound healing and scar formation in plastic surgery have a huge esthetic impact and because of this, HBOT draws significant attention from cosmetic companies as well [5, 6].

Next argument for HBOT is that recent publications suggest its beneficial role in neurodegenerative diseases, such as multiple sclerosis [6]. Latest treatment options, for instance mesenchymal stem cell (MSC) implantation, also comprise hyperbaric treatment or preconditioning. Therapeutic potency of MSC improves after hyperbaric modification [8–10].

Other clinical applications of HBOT are severe anemia, crush injury and gas embolism, necrotizing fasciitis, osteomyelitis, brain abscesses and delayed radiation injury. Evidence is lacking in application for Parkinson's disease and autism.

In vitro models of HBOT utilize wide range of cell lines and tissue cultures [9]. HBOT can be combined with modification of cell culture circumstances, for example, adding active drugs, small molecules, growth factors or signaling drives, according to the focus of interest of the study protocol. Mostly, hyperbaric treatments are applied in parallel with normoxic and hypoxic conditions to implicate useful comparative data. Importantly, *in vitro* models have severe limitations as they are not capable to model the whole pathology and tissue characteristics treated with HBOT. *In vitro* models usually follow the clinical protocols of HBOT, regarding timing and incubation periods [10]. In this chapter, altered oxygen levels of human endothelial cell cultures, fibroblasts cultures, human MSC and pluripotent stem cell (PSC) cultures will be discussed, mirroring the effects of HBOT on angiogenesis, blood clotting, wound healing and future cell therapy/tissue engineering issues.

2. Altered levels of oxygen in cell cultures

2.1. Methods of altered oxygen levels in cell culture

Hyperbaric oxygen treatment of cell cultures can be performed in hyperbaric cell culture chamber *in vitro*. Hyperbaric chambers are available commercially and offer sterile cell culture conditions for short- or long-term maintenance. Cells are usually exposed to 100% oxygen in these chambers; however, some studies comprise 98% oxygen and 2% CO_2 [11]. The level of hyperbaric pressure varies between 1.5 and 3 atmospheres absolute. Compression and decompression times may be applied according to focus of interest and study protocol. Standardization of basic research protocols is key to move the latest investigations with HBOT to clinical translation. Besides HBOT, oxygen levels may be modified for normal or low oxygen (hypoxic) conditions. For normoxic treatment (21% O_2), general cell culture conditions are suitable (5% CO_2, 95% normal air). Hypoxia can be induced by replacing oxygen with nitrogen in cell culture incubators. Mostly, 5 or 10% oxygen levels are investigated in cell culture studies. The same cell culture media and culturing surface can be used in altered oxygen levels, HBOT and in normal conditions [12, 13].

More detailed studies comprise direct quantification of oxygen consumption levels in cellular cultures. These data provide information also on metabolomics status, indirectly on cellular energy homeostasis and metabolic activity of the investigated cultures [14]. Planning studies with direct measurement of oxygen consumption levels enable investigation of cellular function keep with oxygen consumption.

2.2. Endothelial cells, angiogenesis

It is widely accepted that endothelial cells play a key role in a number of important physiological conditions and in pathological steps as well. Endothelial functions comprise regulation of blood flow via regulating vascular tone, vasodilation or vasocontraction. Furthermore, endothelial cells and their expressed factors are cornerstones in initiating or inhibiting platelet activation and blood clotting. Next role is inflammatory mechanisms, white blood cell rolling and diapedesis. Furthermore, special sites of endothelial barriers are the blood–brain barrier, the renal glomeruli and the portal endothelial cells. All these sites have complex barrier and gating functions. All endothelial functions can be modeled *in vitro* and may be investigated and modified via changing oxygen levels or by application of HBOT for cultures.

Additionally, endothelial cells regulate and are involved in embryonic vasculogenesis and somatic angiogenesis as well. Neo-angiogenesis is a key pathological step in tumorous proliferation and metastases development as well. To fulfill these tasks, endothelial cells produce and secrete wide range of angiogenesis-related proteins and small molecules. These may be investigated on gene expression or on the translational (protein) level.

Endothelial cells are keen to proliferate *in vitro,* wide range of cell lines and primary cultures are also available commercially. Widely used endothelial lines *in vitro* are the human umbilical vein endothelial cells (HUVEC), the human coronary arterial endothelial cell (HCAEC), capillary endothelial cells and others from human and animal sources as well. Arterial and venous endothelial cells can be divided via cell surface markers and genotype properties. Arterial and venous endothelial phenotypes differ also *in vitro* because the arterial and venous vessels have largely different functional tasks *in vivo*. As an example, arterial endothelial cells are the major regulators of peripheral vascular resistance, while venous capillary endothelium is the localization for white blood cells' rolling and diapedesis [15]. Furthermore, venous endothelial junctions are thinner, and vessels have greater compliance. Interestingly, arterial and venous plasticity exists *in vitro,* for example, HUVEC surprisingly express arterial markers *in vitro* [16].

Endothelial cells may be cultured in universal cell culturing dishes, on various surfaces, for example, gelatin, fibronectin, collagen and laminin. Common endothelial cell culture media are DMEM and endothelial growth media. To enhance proliferation of mature cells or differentiation from stem cells, a range of growth factors and cytokines can be applied to culture. Important characteristic of mature endothelial cells *in vitro* is the contact inhibition of proliferation [17]. This means that endothelial cells are only capable to proliferate in monolayer trend and grow onto free surfaces. Once the monolayer surface is full-grown, endothelial cell refuses to proliferate *in vitro*.

When investigating endothelial culture, most important *in vitro* characteristics of endothelial cells are the following: phenotype appearance (cobblestone pattern), expression of endothelial specific cell surface markers (CD31, CD144, vascular-endothelial cadherin), acetylated low-density-lipoprotein uptake, tube formation on Matrigel surface and wound healing assay [18]. During passage mechanisms, usually trypsin-based enzymatic digestion is utilized.

Interestingly, these endothelial characteristics were studied in HBOT circumstances as well (**Figure 1**). The morphology of adult somatic endothelial cells in response to HBOT did not change. They retained their cobblestone pattern after HBOT [19]. Importantly, viability of endothelial cells improved after 24 h of HBOT. Increase in viability was related to increase in proliferative capacity as well. Nitric oxide synthase (NOS) has pivotal role in endothelium-dependent vasoactive actions. Role of HBOT treatment was investigated on gene expression levels and on protein levels of primary microvascular capillary endothelial cell cultures. The mechanisms of actions needed further investigations, briefly NOS levels were increased in genomic and protein levels as well [20]. In-depth micro-array analyses of microvascular endothelial cells' genome proved huge impact of HBOT on angiogenesis-related gene expressions [21]. In these studies, HBOT dramatically increased tube formation capacity of endothelial cells on Matrigel [22]. Other studies also proved that HBOT had significant effects on endothelial cells tube formation and migration capacity. Short-term (6–8 h) HBOT treatment resulted in increased migration capacity and enhanced tube formation also by length and density of the network [20]. Ingenuity pathway analyses of the microarray expression data proved top responder's genes for HBOT. These top responder genes were all related to cell-matrix adhesion and matrix degradation processes. The analyses further provided quantitative data on the absolute percentage of endothelial cells that have a specific modulation, such as cellular growth and proliferation 41%, cell death 39%, gene expression 34%, cell morphology 16% and cell cycle 13% [23].

In angiogenesis, main initiative steps are orchestrated by VEGF. Both by sprouting and intussusceptive angiogenesis, the main drive brings activation by VEGF isoforms and their receptors. These VEGFs set communication between tip, phalanx, stalk cells and pericytes [24]. Many other endothelial growth factors and small molecules take part in this process, for example, fibroblast growth factor, epidermal growth factor, insulin-like growth factor, Ephrins and Ephrin receptors, angiopoietin-1, angiopoietin-2 and their receptors [25]. Furthermore, the complex regulatory pathway of the renin-angiotensin-aldosteron system also interacts with vascular mechanism. Amount of secreted angiogenesis-related factors can be measured *in vitro* from cell culture supernatants and from cell lysates via proteolysis. Interestingly, angiogenesis-related steps and molecules may also play a role in chronic tinnitus, which tends to be a future disease to be treated with HBOT [26].

http://dx.doi.org/10.5772/intechopen.75378

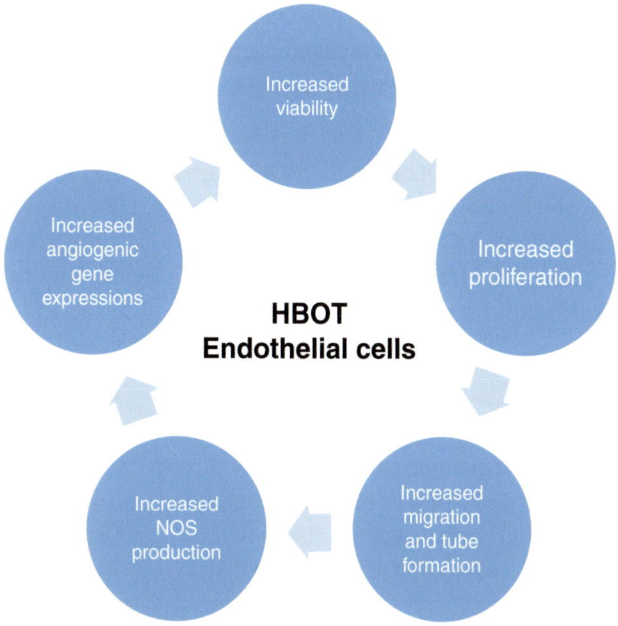

Figure 1. Angiogenesis-related effects of HBOT on endothelial cells.

2.3. Endothelial cells, blood clotting

Besides angiogenesis, orchestrating of blot clotting is a foremost characteristic of endothelial cells. Importantly, altered oxygen circumstances can change endothelial responsiveness, platelet activation and clotting mechanisms. Tissue plasminogen activator is the most powerful enzyme to catalyze thrombin via activating plasminogen to cleave thrombin. Interesting *in vitro* studies proved that HBOT has the potential to modify tissue plasminogen activator secretion from endothelial cells [27]. The changes observed would be clinically significant and beneficial, even more, considering advantageous effects of HBOT on blood-brain barrier function. Others also measured tissue plasminogen activator in combination with plasminogen activator-inhibitor from endothelial supernatants, immediately after HBOT treatment. Surprisingly, both peptides were significantly increased after short-term HBOT. Increased expression was observed immediately after the HBOT and remained also significantly higher at 6 h follow-up of treatment [28].

Additionally, beside regulating endothelial cells-related clot cytokines, HBOT also had notable effects on platelet activity and function as well. Interestingly, platelets responded to HBOT in a manner that their NOS secretion increased significantly [29]. This phenomenon can have significant effects on platelet clotting and thrombus formation as well [9]; however detailed understanding is warranted.

Some human clinical studies investigated platelet count and activity after HBOT and surprisingly found no significant difference before and after HBOT [30]. *In vitro* models often use altered levels and timing of HBOT and most *in vitro* effects are not directly translatable to *in vivo* human responses. For instance, platelet rich plasma in experimental circumstances improved after HBOT and had more advantageous effects in a pro-inflammatory, pro-thrombotic area *in vivo* [31]. Mostly, these mechanisms act differently in whole bodies *in vivo*.

Some studies concluded that HBOT may also have disadvantageous effects *in vivo*, if the timing and longevity of treatment is not optimal. Interestingly, in experimental setup, HBOT was able to modify renal erythropoietin production. Disadvantageous results came after HBOT was released and rebound effects ameliorated normal erythropoietin levels. Thus, renal tissue failed to cope with sudden and frequent changes in oxygen levels. The observed results were unrelated to circadian rhythm of erythropoietin production [32].

Point-of-care whole blood and platelet clot analyzer systems also brought disappointing data. Some of these ex vivo analyses proved that short-term HBOT may initiate *in vitro* steps which are characteristics of a disseminated intravascular coagulation (DIC) [33]. DIC is a severe, life threating condition, comprising both pro-thrombotic and not-clotting elements, resulting in a severe clinical case, when blood is unable to clot, but small capillaries are impaired by thrombi. In response to HBOT, an increase in the maximum clot firmness and thrombo-elastic component in clot firmness was depicted (**Figure 2**) [33].

2.4. Endothelial cells, barrier and inflammation

Nitric oxide (NO) is one of the most important factors released by endothelial cells. NO plays a pivotal role in setting vascular tone and regulating blood pressure, via arterioles. On the venous circuit site, NO also has vasodilatory effects, thus is a major vasoactive factor at the site of white blood cells diapedesis and extravasation. Beside these, NO also counteracts with angiogenic activities.

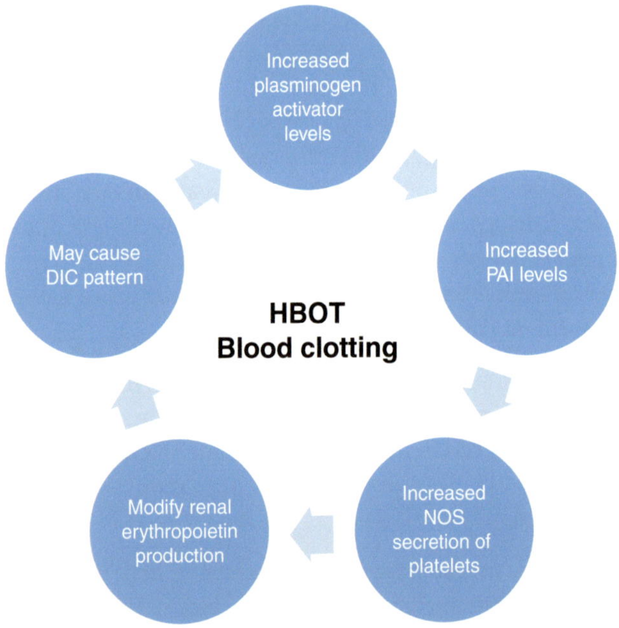

Figure 2. Effects of HBOT on blood clotting. PAI: plasminogen activator inhibitor, DIC: disseminated intravasulcar coagulation.

Interestingly, blood-brain barrier function of endothelial cells can also be modeled and investigated *in vitro*. This very special and crucial endothelial site of the human body is key in pharmacological interventions and critically ill patients. Altered oxygen levels have different effects on blood-brain barrier. It is widely believed that decreased oxygen availability, for example, ischemic attack of the brain, has huge impact on the existence and proper function of blood-brain barrier. In stroke, blood-brain barrier lacks its gating function and medications may have altered neurological side effects as well.

In the in vitro model of blood-brain barrier, brain microvascular endothelial cells can be cultured and trans-endothelial electric potential, as a measure of barrier function, can be evaluated in different oxygen circumstances [34]. Mainly cell interactions, tight junctions and endothelial-pericyte interactions are damaged in blood-brain barrier dysfunction. Cell adhesion molecules are often investigated *in vitro* as well. Endothelial and pericyte co-cultures (e.g., insert plate) offer studying communication between these cellular compartments [35].

In co-culture, cellular models of endothelial interactions with white blood cells were also observed. White blood cells' diapedesis, rolling and pooling in microcirculation are the determinants of local inflammatory responses. Attenuating these would have dramatic therapeutic effects, for example, in chronic, not-healing wounds. Neutrophils' adhesion to endothelial cells was reversed and delayed in HBOT circumstances [36]. The underlying molecular mechanism was mainly the reduced expression of neutrophil-endothelial adhesion molecule, ICAM-1. As a result of low neutrophil adhesion, local levels of ROS were also decreased [36].

Further studies proved that HBOT may have direct effects on endothelial gene expression as well. HCAEC modified their angiogenesis-related gene expression, shortly after HBOT. Short-term HBOT (4–6 h) resulted in increased TNF-α secretion from HCAEC. Related to this, HBOT also modified expression of a range of peptides and small molecular, which have strong role in glucose metabolism and inflammatory reactions as well [20]. Additionally, all of these mechanisms were also linked to altered expressions of certain kinases and altered phosphorylation status. These were related to visceral fat accumulation, atherosclerosis, inflammation and increased cardiovascular risk. Remarkable results proved that HBOT also have metabolomics effects on treated endothelial cells. Short-term HBOT altered glucose uptake in HCEAC. These key results showed that metabolomics disturbances may also be modified under HBOT circumstances, which has key message to future therapeutic human applications [20].

Interestingly, HBOT had robust effect on inflammation-related cytokine expression, for example, level of anti-inflammatory angiogenin decreased, while the level of pro-inflammatory cytokines (IL-6 and IL-8) significantly decreased in response to HBOT. This *in vitro* model was established from and *in vivo* septic small animal model. Endothelial cells from septic and control rats were cultures and inflammatory cytokines were measured from endothelial supernatants [37]. Others also showed significant decrease in pro-inflammatory cytokines, such as TNF-α following HBOT [38].

Latest *in vitro* studies demonstrated that hypoxic damage of blood-brain barrier may be reversed via HBOT [34]. Hypoxia induced cellular endothelial fragmentation and impair of cell adhesion molecular. On the contrary, HBOT after hypoxia was able to attenuate the effects and improve cellular junctions [34]. These data have very important message to clinical trials, as HBOT may have undistinguishable role in stroke treatment in the acute clinical phase (**Figure 3**) [39].

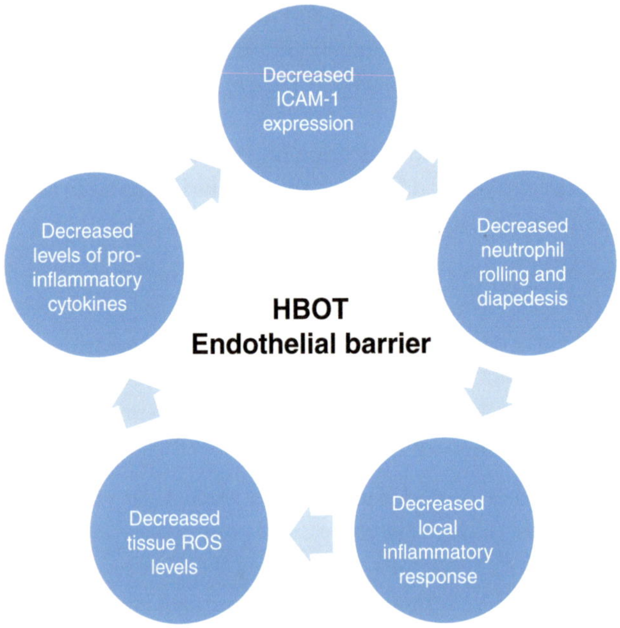

Figure 3. Effects of HBOT on endothleial barrier and local inflammatory reactions.

2.5. Fibroblasts, wound healing

Fibroblasts are easy to culture and maintain. They have high proliferative capacity and low maintenance circumstances. They grow in any cell culture media, mostly in fibroblast growth media or DMEM. They adhere to plastic surfaces or to any additional, for example, gelatin or fibronectin. Interestingly, fibroblasts proliferative from skin biopsy samples *in vitro* as well. Fibroblasts have rod-shaped, elongated phenotype in culture. Usually they proliferate in monolayer; however, contact inhibition of growth is not as prominent as it is by endothelial cells [40].

Chronic, not-healing wounds are major challenge in dermatology, surgery and plastic surgery [4, 7]. These wounds have valuable impact on diabetic and cardiovascular patients' quality of life. Furthermore, these wounds often become infected or colonized with resistant species, for example, MRSA [41]. Mechanisms of action in these chronic wounds include reactive oxygen species, chronic inflammation and chronic ischemia [42]. The connective tissue, extracellular matrices are also affected and hyper-oxidant status seems to be the common clue behind non-healing. Growth and proliferation of fibroblasts are often impaired due to aforementioned pathological mechanisms. Thus, fibroblasts offer platform to monitor cellular events on one important component of these wounds. *In vitro* studies are suitable to monitor effects of altered oxygen levels, especially focusing on cytokine release, apoptosis and leukocyte activation.

In vitro studies proved that HBOT on ischemic wound tissue increased the activity of superoxide-dismutase (SOD) enzyme, which is known to be one of the most potent enzymes acting against ROS species-related harm [43]. Interestingly, *in vivo* studies on small animal models of chronic ulcers also proved significant effects of matrix-metalloproteinases (MMP) in the chronic ongoing

http://dx.doi.org/10.5772/intechopen.75378

damage. Placing the animals in HBOT and treating them resulted in increased MMP inhibitor activity and in parallel the tissue damage, cellular apoptosis and necrosis decreased [44].

HBOT has a significant effect on the growth of fibroblast cultures. HBOT in increasing pressure and time interval had advantageous effects on the proliferation of fibroblast cultures, suggesting beneficial effects in wound healing steps as well [45]. Parallel with timing and pressure of HBOT, cell numbers increased as well [45]. Additionally, HBOT increased tube formation of endothelial and fibroblast co-cultures [20]. In a wound healing assay, *in vitro*, significant increase was observed after HBOT treatment [22]. Linking to previous clues, HBOT also increases collagen proliferation [22], parallel with beneficial effects on fibroblast growth, and thus all together, HBOT has a beneficial effect on extracellular matrix proliferation, growth and structure [20]. Furthermore, recent experiments proved the increase of fibroblast proliferation and growth also *in vitro* and *in vivo* in epidural fibrous tissue. Mechanisms of action behind these were downregulation of canonical TGF-β and interleukin pathways, which were responsible for maintaining fibroblasts' viability and proliferation (**Figure 4**) [46].

TGF-β is also involved in uncontrolled scar formation, known as keloid scars [47]. Keloid scars contain highly proliferative fibroblasts and connective tissues, which cause significant biomechanical and esthetic problems on affected skins. HBOT were successful to reduce TFG-β levels in these keloids and interestingly proliferation of keloid scar was postponed in response to HBOT [48]. The regulatory steps are not yet characterized in detail, and further investigation is needed to understand the process [49].

In vitro models for burned skins also exist; however, modeling the complex mechanisms of local and systemic response to severe burn and demonstrating and measuring accurately the cytokine storm *in vitro* are almost impossible. Interesting *in vitro* model for burned skin evolved ex vivo available burned skin tissues [50]. Recently, HBOT has been emerged for the treatment of chronic burn-related wounds as inflammatory cytokine release was decreased and bacterial viability also decreased in wound [34, 35]. Burn models proved hyperemia (improved microcirculation) and reduced size of the burned lesions after HBOT of burn wounds [53]. Additionally, fluid homeostasis of burned wounds was also altered beneficially after HBOT [51, 52]. Intercellular edema decreased after HBOT, resulting in better microcirculatory responses and increased debris elimination [54].

2.6. Mesenchymal and pluripotent stem cells, cell therapy and tissue engineering aspects

MSC and other cell types such as the pluripotent stem cells have huge potential for cell therapy and tissue engineering in various diseases. Recently, most clinical trials in cardiovascular field have been performed with MSC or MSC-derivatives [55]. Furthermore, cardiovascular derivatives of pluripotent stem cells are promising tools to differentiate new cardiovascular cells and to build cardiovascular tissue. Latest tissue engineering methods comprise biodegradable matrices combined with cellular building blocks.

MSC and PSC behave and differentiate altered in normal hypoxic or in hyperbaric oxygen conditions PSC studies concluded that altered oxygen levels may mimic in utero conditions

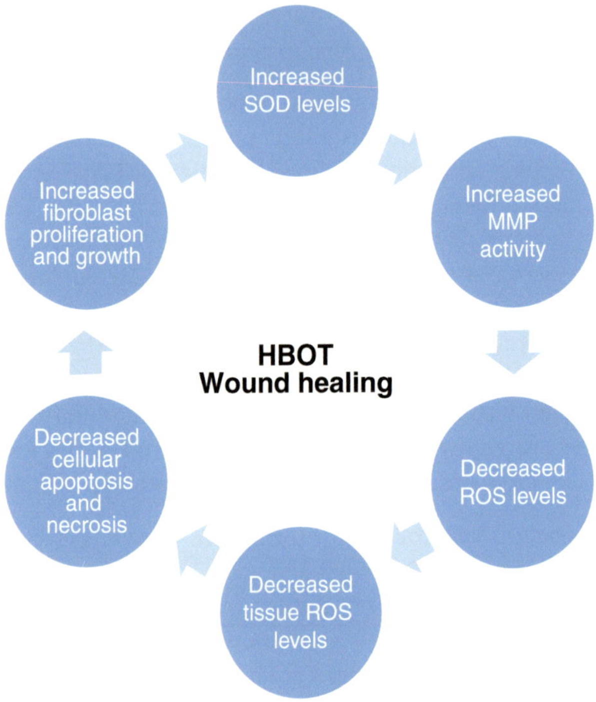

Figure 4. Effects of HBOT on wound healing and fibroblasts SOD: superoxide dismutase, MMP: matrix-metalloproteinase, ROS: reactive oxygen species.

better and thus may initiate differentiation potency [56]. Latest state-of-the-art molecular biology protocols comprise epigenetic or genetic modifications for example reprogramming and CRISPR/Cas9 genome editing technique [57, 58]. These are often utilized parallel with altered oxygen levels. Signaling steps related to these mechanisms also changed including MAP kinases [44].

MSCs are multipotent stem cells which by definition have the potency to differentiate into cartilage bone muscle tendon ligament and fat tissue. MSC can be characterized via cell surface markers: they widely express CD73, CD90 and CD105 but do not express CD11, CD14, CD19, CD34 and CD45 [57]. They are easy to culture adhere to plastic and most cell culture surfaces and can proliferate in MSC media and others as well. By directed differentiation they can differentiate into chondrogenic osteogenic myogenic and adipogenous linage [57]. It is debated if mature cardiomyocytes can derive from MSC.

Hypoxic preconditioning is currently being investigated also in human clinical trials as a protective mechanism of ischemia-reperfusion injury in the ischemic myocardium [59]. Related to this, ischemic preconditioning is being evaluated in the *in vitro* setting and in clinical trials. Recently, MSC were the most robust players in cardiovascular cell therapy trials. For instance, the CHART-1 clinical trial involved hundreds of patients suffering from chronic ischemic heart failure. Cardiopoietic cells, derived from MSC, were implanted endomyocardially.

Despite huge promises, the CHART-1 trial failed to reach primary composite endpoint and cell implantation did not improve functional status of the patients [38–40, 60, 61]. The pre-implanted cells received a growth factor cocktail, but none-of oxygen level modification was performed during pretreatment [62]. Earlier studies proved that hypoxic preconditioning of MSC increases their secretion of pro-angiogenic, anti-fibrotic, anti-apoptotic secretome, which are known as the paracrine mechanism [63]. Some of these trials comprised temporary anoxia as well [64]. Beside hypoxic pretreatment, other studies aimed hyperbaric pretreatment of regenerative studies [65]. Preconditioning in HBOT circumstances had advantageous effects on neuronal cells as well [65]. *In vitro* part of small animals' trials proved that HBOT can induce hypoxia tolerability of spinal neurons. The mechanisms of actions behind these beneficial effects were metabolic coping, especially altered glucose homeostasis [66]. Thus, these experiments underpinned that HBOT has direct effect on metabolomics and energy homeostasis of cellular compartments, as different oxygen levels await altered metabolic actions [66].

HBOT in MSC resulted in increased proliferative capacity of the cells when compared to those MSC treated in normal oxygen circumstances [11, 29]. In this study, secretome of MSC was evaluated via the ELISA method and levels of BDNF were investigated. This peptide has pivotal role in neurodegenerative diseases but also reported to play a role in salvage mechanisms of the central nervous system after a cardiac arrest [67]. BDNF secretion of MSC significantly increased after HBOT treatment, but was also improved in hypoxia [45]. These results widely clue if normal oxygen levels are suitable to culture and maintain MSC and their derivatives. Further cell therapy trials are needed to standardize cell culture protocols, because recent variations disable direct comparative analyses.

Endothelial progenitor cells [68] are circulating in blood and released from bone marrow. Some studies outline their potential biomarker role for ischemic cardiovascular conditions, as far as their level is increased in acute myocardial infarction and chronic hind-limb ischemia [69]. Endothelial progenitor cells may also have therapeutic effects and phase II/III clinical trials aim boosting them by external infusion of activating factors [70]. An activator drive of these circulating progenitor cells could also be HBOT [71]. Repeated HBOT resulted in significant release of circulating CD34 positive progenitor cells in the peripheral blood. The mechanisms were NOS dependent [71].

If directed differentiation is aimed to be supported, MSC may be cultured in HBOT circumstances. Interestingly, HBOT enhanced osteogenic differentiation of MSC, which *in vitro* description was further proved via *in vivo* proof-of-concept studies as well [11]. Interestingly, metabolic activities, especially calcium influx and exchange, were also modulated by HBOT in MSC. HBOT increased the activity of calcium homeostasis, which is key for osteoblasts via proliferation and bone formation [11].

Pluripotent stem cells are sensitive cell cultures *in vitro*. Their maintenance requires special techniques and expertise in the field. Pluripotent cells form pluripotent cell clusters *in vitro*. They require special maintenance pluripotent stem cell media. Through passaging, spontaneously differentiated cells have to be picked and removed from culture. Recently, enzymatic passage became more advantageous than mechanical breaking of pluripotent colonies.

Pluripotent stem cell maintenance and differentiation are new and difficult cell culture techniques. These involve monolayer or three-dimensional/cell suspension culture as well. Pluripotent stem cell may be cultured on feeder layer of feeder-free surface on biomatrices. The pluripotent stem cells themselves have excellent viability and proliferative capacity in normal oxygen circumstances [72]. Additionally, they are immortal and can continuously proliferate in pluripotent state. Reasonably, most study protocols emphasize the importance of altered oxygen levels, once differentiation steps are in progress. After differentiation, steps are initiated altered oxygen levels usually increase the yield of developed cells and increase functional activity, for example, insulin secretion of beta cells, derived from pluripotent cells [14].

Pluripotent stem cells proliferate in low-oxygen levels in utero. It is also agreed that MSC have low oxygen circumstances *in vivo* in the bone marrow niche. Taking these into consideration, *in vitro* culture of the cells in normal oxygen circumstances is out of their normal niche. Interestingly, all of these cell types improved performance in therapeutic potential when cultured in hypoxic environment [45]. MSC improved angiogenesis-related gene expressions and protein expressions in hypoxia, furthermore implanting them into various *in vivo* models of ischemia resulted in better outcomes [73].

HBOT would have a significant role in tissue engineering and preconditioning the engineered construct *in vitro*, before *in vivo* transplantation. As an example, tissue engineered mucosa were further developed in HBOT. The mucosal cells enhanced expression of angiogenesis-related factor (e.g., VEGF, FGF and HGF) [74]. Enhanced angiogenesis by mucosal tissue may be beneficial for graft homing and retention.

Wide range of differentiation protocols exist, which aim improving the number of cardiovascular derivatives after the differentiation steps. These are increasing in endothelial cell and cardiovascular cells as well. With endothelial cells, recent protocols reached about 50% differentiation yield. Latest studies aim hypoxia as a diver to mesodermal and then to endothelial lineage specification [75].

3. Conclusion

In conclusion, HBOT is an interesting novel medical tool with wide range of therapeutic potential.

In vitro cellular models utilize different HBOT protocols and need to be standardized to bring translatable data to clinicians.

This chapter outlined that HBOT increases endothelial and fibroblast viability and proliferation *in vitro*. Furthermore, tube formation and wound healing assay improved in response to HBOT. HBOT has significant effects on endothelial-related blot-clotting and platelet mechanisms as well. Furthermore, HBOT decreases ROS-related harm in not-healing wound model and improves blood-brain barrier after ischemic event in *in vitro* model. In new therapeutic promises, the stem cells would also benefit from HBOT in maintenance, proliferation and tissue engineering aspects as well.

http://dx.doi.org/10.5772/intechopen.75378

Conflict of interest

The author declares no conflict of interest.

Abbreviations

CO	carbon monoxide
CO_2	carbon dioxide
HBOT	hyperbaric oxygen treatment
NO	nitric oxide
NOS	nitric oxide synthase
MRSA	methicillin-resistant *Staphylococcus aureus*
MSC	mesenchymal stem cells
PSC	pluripotent stem cells
ROS	reactive oxygen species
SOD	superoxide-dismutase

Author details

Edit Gara

Address all correspondence to: gara.edit@med.semmelweis-univ.hu

Semmelweis University, Budapest, Hungary

References

[1] Cevik NG, Orhan N, Yilmaz CU, Arican N, Ahishali B, Kucuk M, Kaya M, Toklu AS. The effects of hyperbaric airand hyperbaric oxygen on blood-brain barrier integrity in rats. Brain Res. 2013 Sep 19;**1531**:113-121

[2] Weaver LK et al. Hyperbaric oxygen for acute carbon monoxide poisoning. The New England Journal of Medicine. 2002;**347**(14):1057-1067

[3] Löndahl M, Katzman P, Nilsson A, Hammarlund C. Hyperbaric oxygen therapy facilitates healing of chronic foot ulcers in patients with diabetes. Diabetes Care. 2010; **33**(5):998-1003

[4] Stoekenbroek RM, Santema TB, Legemate DA, Ubbink DT, Van Den Brink A, Koelemay MJW. Hyperbaric oxygen for the treatment of diabetic foot ulcers: A systematic review. European Journal of Vascular and Endovascular Surgery. 2014;**47**(6):647-655

[5] Hunter S, Langemo DK, Anderson J, Hanson D, Thompson P. Hyperbaric oxygen therapy for chronic wounds. Advances in Skin & Wound Care. 2010;**23**(3):116-119

[6] GMG. Hyperbaric oxygen treatment (HBOT) in neurology. Journal of the Neurological Sciences. 2009;**285**:S22

[7] Gottrup F. Oxygen in wound healing and infection. World Journal of Surgery. 2004; **28**(3):312-315

[8] Cohen JA. Mesenchymal stem cell transplantation in multiple sclerosis. Journal of the Neurological Sciences. 2013;**333**(1-2):43-49

[9] Thom SR et al. Vasculogenic stem cell mobilization and wound recruitment in diabetic patients: Increased cell number and intracellular regulatory protein content associated with hyperbaric oxygen therapy. Wound Repair and Regeneration. 2011;**19**(2):149-161

[10] Kraitsy K et al. Repetitive long-term hyperbaric oxygen treatment (HBOT) administered after experimental traumatic brain injury in rats induces significant remyelination and a recovery of sensorimotor function. PLoS One. 2014;**9**(5):e97750

[11] Lin S-S et al. Hyperbaric oxygen promotes osteogenic differentiation of bone marrow stromal cells by regulating Wnt3a/β-catenin signaling--an *in vitro* and *in vivo* study. Stem Cell Research. 2014;**12**(1):260-274

[12] André-Lévigne D, Modarressi A, Pignel R, Bochaton-Piallat ML, Pittet-Cuénod B. Hyperbaric oxygen therapy promotes wound repair in ischemic and hyperglycemic conditions, increasing tissue perfusion and collagen deposition. Wound Repair and Regeneration. 2016;**24**(6):954-965

[13] Philippeos C, Hughes RD, Dhawan A, Mitry RR. Introduction to cell culture. Methods in Molecular Biology. 2012;**806**:1-13

[14] Cechin S et al. Influence of *in vitro* and *in vivo* oxygen modulation on beta cell differentiation from human embryonic stem cells. Stem Cells Translational Medicine. 2014; **3**:277-289

[15] De Mey JG, Vanhoutte PM. Heterogeneous behavior of the canine arterial and venous wall. Importance of the endothelium. Circulation Research. 1982;**51**(4):439-447

[16] Sivarapatna A, Ghaedi M, Le AV, Mendez JJ, Qyang Y, Niklason LE. Arterial specification of endothelial cells derived from human induced pluripotent stem cells in a biomimetic flow bioreactor. Biomaterials. 2015;**53**:621-633

[17] Lampugnani MG et al. Contact inhibition of VEGF-induced proliferation requires vascular endothelial cadherin, β-catenin, and the phosphatase DEP-1/CD148. The Journal of Cell Biology. 2003;**161**(4):793-804

http://dx.doi.org/10.5772/intechopen.75378

[18] Reed DM et al. Morphology and vasoactive hormone profiles from endothelial cells derived from stem cells of different sources. Biochemical and Biophysical Research Communications. 2014;**455**(3-4)

[19] Xu X et al. Endothelial nitric oxide synthase expression is progressively increased in primary cerebral microvascular endothelial cells during hyperbaric oxygen exposure. Oxidative Medicine and Cellular Longevity. 2009;**2**(1):7-13

[20] Wang B-W, Lin C-M, Wu G-J, Shyu K-G. Tumor necrosis factor-α enhances hyperbaric oxygen-induced visfatin expression via JNK pathway in human coronary arterial endothelial cells. Journal of Biomedical Science. 2011;**18**:27

[21] Montecorboli U, Annese T, Marinaccio C, Ribatti D. Angiogenesis and hyperbaric oxygen in the chick embryo chorioallantoic membrane. The International Journal of Developmental Biology. 2015;**59**(10-12):461-464

[22] Godman CA, Chheda KP, Hightower LE, Perdrizet G, Shin D-G, Giardina C. Hyperbaric oxygen induces a cytoprotective and angiogenic response in human microvascular endothelial cells. Cell Stress Chaperones. 2010;**15**(4):431-442

[23] Godman C, Chheda K, Hightower L, Perdrizet G, Shin D-G, Giardina C. Hyperbaric oxygen induces a cytoprotective and angiogenic response in human microvascular endothelial cells. Cell Stress & Chaperones. 2010 Jul;**15**(4):431-442

[24] Ribatti D, Crivellato E. 'Sprouting angiogenesis', a reappraisal. Developmental Biology. 2012;**372**(2):157-165

[25] De Val S et al. Transcriptional control of endothelial cell development. Arteriosclerosis, Thrombosis, and Vascular Biology. 2013;**99**(11):13-19

[26] Jung S, Wermker K, Poetschik H, Ziebura T, Kleinheinz J. The impact of hyperbaric oxygen therapy on serological values of vascular endothelial growth factor (VEGF) and basic fibroblast growth factor (bFGF). Head & Face Medicine. 2010;**6**(1):29

[27] Su EJ et al. Activation of PDGF-CC by tissue plasminogen activator impairs blood-brain barrier integrity during ischemic stroke. Nature Medicine. 2008;**14**(7):731-737

[28] Tjärnström J, Holmdahl L, Arnell P, Falkenberg M, Risberg B. Treatment with hyperbaric oxygen affects endothelial cell fibrinolysis. The European Journal of Surgery. 1999;**165**(9):834-838

[29] Polom W, Klejnotowska A, Matuszewski M, Sicko Z, Markuszewski M, Krajkal K. Hyperbaric oxygen therapy (HBOT) in case of hemorrhagic cystitis after radiotherapy. Central European Journal of Urology. 2012;**65**(4):200-203

[30] Thom SR, Fisher D, Stubbs JM. Platelet function in humans is not altered by hyperbaric oxygen therapy. Undersea & Hyperbaric Medicine. 2006;**33**(2):81-83

[31] Yümün G et al. Effects of hyperbaric oxygen therapy combined with plateletrich plasma on diabetic wounds: An experimental rat model. Archives Medical Science. 2016;**12**(6):1370-1376

[32] Balestra C. Serum erythropoietin levels in healthy humans after a short period of normobaric and hyperbaric oxygen breathing: The 'normobaric oxygen paradox. Journal of Applied Physiology. 2006;**100**(2):512-518

[33] Monaca E et al. Assessment of hemostaseologic alterations induced by hyperbaric oxygen therapy using point-of-care analyzers. Undersea & Hyperbaric Medicine. 2014;**41**(1):17-26

[34] Hao L et al. Hyperbaric oxygen preconditioning ameliorates blood-brain barrier damage induced by hypoxia through modulation of tight junction proteins in an *in vitro* model. Croatian Medical Journal. 2016;**57**(1):51-57

[35] Tarallo S, Beltramo E, Berrone E, Porta M. Human pericyte-endothelial cell interactions in co-culture models mimicking the diabetic retinal microvascular environment. Acta Diabetologica. 2012;**49**:S141-S151

[36] Kendall AC, Whatmore JL, Winyard PG, Smerdon GR, Eggleton P. Hyperbaric oxygen treatment reduces neutrophil-endothelial adhesion in chronic wound conditions through S-nitrosation. Wound Repair and Regeneration. 2013;**21**(6):860-868

[37] Avtan SM et al. The effects of hyperbaric oxygen therapy on blood-brain barrier permeability in septic rats. Brain Research. 2011;**1412**:63-72

[38] Kendall AC, Whatmore JL, Harries LW, Winyard PG, Eggleton P, Smerdon GR. Different oxygen treatment pressures alter inflammatory gene expression in human endothelial cells. Undersea & Hyperbaric Medicine. 2013;**40**(2):115-123

[39] Bennett MH, Weibel S, Wasiak J, Schnabel A, French C, Kranke P. Hyperbaric oxygen therapy for acute ischaemic stroke. Cochrane Database of Systematic Reviews. 2014;**11**: 004954

[40] Darby IA, Hewitson TD. Fibroblast differentiation in wound healing and fibrosis. International Review of Cytology. 2007;**257**:143-179

[41] Demling RH, Waterhouse B. The increasing problem of wound bacterial burden and infection in acute and chronic soft-tissue wounds caused by methicillin-resistant *Staphylococcus aureus*. Journal of Burns and Wounds. 2007;**7**(1554-0766 (Electronic)):e8

[42] Frykberg RG, Banks J. Challenges in the treatment of chronic wounds. Advances in Wound Care. 2015;**4**(9):560-582

[43] Parabucki AB et al. Hyperbaric oxygenation alters temporal expression pattern of superoxide dismutase 2 after cortical stab injury in rats. Croatian Medical Journal. 2012; **53**(6):586-597

[44] Zhang Q, Gould LJ. Hyperbaric oxygen reduces matrix metalloproteinases in ischemic wounds through a redox-dependent mechanism. The Journal of Investigative Dermatology. 2014;**134**(1):237-246

[45] Schulze J et al. Effect of hyperbaric oxygen on BDNF-release and neuroprotection: Investigations with human mesenchymal stem cells and genetically modified NIH3T3 fibroblasts as putative cell therapeutics. PLoS One. 2017;**12**(5):0178182

[46] Lv P, Zhao J, Su W, Liang X, Zhang K. An experimental novel study: Hyperbaric oxygen treatment on reduction of epidural fibrosis via down-regulation of collagen deposition, IL-6, and TGF-β1. European Journal of Orthopaedic Surgery and Traumatology. 2015;**25**:53-58

[47] Babu M, Diegelmann R, Oliver N. Keloid fibroblasts exhibit an altered response to TGF-β. The Journal of Investigative Dermatology. 1992;**99**(5):650-655

[48] Al-Attar A, Mess S, Thomassen JM, Kauffman CL, Davison SP. Keloid pathogenesis and treatment. Plastic and Reconstructive Surgery. 2006;**117**(1):286-300

[49] Romero-Valdovinos M, Cárdenas-Mejía A, Gutiérrez-Gómez C, Flisser A, Kawa-Karasik S, Ortiz-Monasterio F. Keloid skin scars: The influence of hyperbaric oxygenation on fibroblast growth and on the expression of messenger RNA for insulin like growth factor and for transforming growth factor. *In Vitro* Cellular & Developmental Biology – Animal. 2011;**47**(7):421-424

[50] Coolen NA, Vlig M, Van Den Bogaerdt AJ, Middelkoop E, Ulrich MMW. Development of an *in vitro* burn wound model. Wound Repair and Regeneration. 2008;**16**(4):559-567

[51] Elkins-Williams ST, Marston WA, Hultman CS. Management of the Chronic Burn Wound. Clinics in Plastic Surgery. 2017;**44**(3):679-687

[52] Weaver LK. Hyperbaric oxygen in the critically ill. Critical Care Medicine. 2011; **39**(7):1784-1791

[53] Niezgoda JA, Cianci P, Folden BW, Ortega RL, Slade JB, Storrow AB. The effect of hyperbaric oxygen therapy on a burn wound model in human volunteers. Plastic and Reconstructive Surgery. 1997;**99**(6):1620-1625

[54] Nylander G, Nordström H, Eriksson E. Effects of hyperbaric oxygen on oedema formation after a scald burn. Burns. 1984;**10**(3):193-196

[55] Madonna R et al. Position paper of the European Society of Cardiology Working Group Cellular Biology of the heart: Cell-based therapies for myocardial repair and regeneration in ischemic heart disease and heart failure. European Heart Journal. 2016;**37**(23):1789-1798

[56] Joddar B, Ito Y. Artificial niche substrates for embryonic and induced pluripotent stem cell cultures. Journal of Biotechnology. 2013;**168**(2):218-228

[57] Gara E, Molnár AÁ, Merkely B, Földes G. Assessing the therapeutic readiness of stem cells for cardiovascular repair. Expert Opinion on Biological Therapy. 2017

[58] Hou Z et al. Efficient genome engineering in human pluripotent stem cells using Cas9 from Neisseria meningitidis. Proceedings of the National Academy of Sciences of the United States of America. 2013;**110**(39):15644-15649

[59] Hu X et al. Safety and efficacy of intracoronary hypoxia-preconditioned bone marrow mononuclear cell administration for acute myocardial infarction patients: The CHINA-AMI randomized controlled trial. International Journal of Cardiology. 2015;**184**(1):446-451

[60] Bartunek J et al. Cardiopoietic cell therapy for advanced ischaemic heart failure: Results at 39 weeks of the prospective, randomized, double blind, sham-controlled CHART-1 clinical trial. European Heart Journal. 2017;**38**(9):648-660

[61] Teerlink JR et al. Benefit of cardiopoietic mesenchymal stem cell therapy on left ventricular remodelling: Results from the congestive heart failure cardiopoietic regenerative therapy (CHART-1) study. European Journal of Heart Failure. 2017;**19**(11):1520-1529

[62] Bartunek J et al. Congestive heart failure cardiopoietic regenerative therapy (CHART-1) trial design. European Journal of Heart Failure. 2016;**18**(2):160-168

[63] Theus MH et al. *In vitro* hypoxic preconditioning of embryonic stem cells as a strategy of promoting cell survival and functional benefits after transplantation into the ischemic rat brain. Experimental Neurology. 2008;**210**(2):656-670

[64] He A, Jiang Y, Gui C, Sun Y, Li J, Wang J. The antiapoptotic effect of mesenchymal stem cell transplantation on ischemic myocardium is enhanced by anoxic preconditioning. Canadian Journal of Cardiology. 2009;**25**(6):353-358

[65] Kuffler DP. The role of hyperbaric oxygen therapy in enhancing the rate of wound healing with a focus on axon regeneration. Puerto Rico Health Sciences Journal. 2011;**30**(1):35-42

[66] Huang G et al. Hyperbaric oxygen preconditioning induces tolerance against oxidative injury and oxygen-glucose deprivation by up-regulating heat shock protein 32 in rat spinal neurons. PLoS One. 2014;**9**(1):85967

[67] Husson I et al. BDNF-induced white matter neuroprotection and stage-dependent neuronal survival following a neonatal excitotoxic challenge. Cerebral Cortex. 2005; **15**(3):250-261

[68] Thom SR, Bhopale VM, Velazquez OC, Goldstein LJ, Thom LH, Buerk DG. Stem cell mobilization by hyperbaric oxygen. American Journal of Physiology-Heart and Circulatory Physiology. 2006;**290**(4):H1378-H1386

[69] Sen S, McDonald SP, Coates PTH, Bonder CS. Endothelial progenitor cells: Novel biomarker and promising cell therapy for cardiovascular disease. Clinical Science (London, England). 2011;**120**(7):263-283

[70] Pelosi E, Castelli G, Testa U. Endothelial progenitors. Blood Cells, Molecules, and Diseases. 2014;**52**(4):186-194

[71] Pereira LR, Conway DH. Adjunctive hyperbaric oxygen therapy (HBOT) in patients with primary immunodeficiency. The Journal of Allergy and Clinical Immunology. 2015; **135**(2):AB183

[72] Merkely B et al. Signaling via PI3K/FOXO1A pathway modulates formation and survival of human embryonic stem cell-derived endothelial cells. Stem Cells and Development. 2015;**24**(7):869-878

[73] Caplan AI, Correa D. The MSC: An injury drugstore. Cell Stem Cell. 2011;**9**(1):11-15

[74] Tra WMW, Spiegelberg L, Tuk B, Hovius SER, Perez-Amodio S. Hyperbaric oxygen treatment of tissue-engineered mucosa enhances secretion of angiogenic factors *in vitro*. Tissue Engineering. Part A. 2014;**20**(9-10):1523-1530

[75] Vittet D et al. Embryonic stem cells differentiate *in vitro* to endothelial cells through successive maturation steps. Blood. 1996;**88**(9):3424-3431

Chapter 6

Mechanisms of HBO-Induced Vascular Functional Changes in Diabetic Animal Models

Ivana Jukic, Mihael Mišir, Martina Mihalj,
Zrinka Mihaljevic, Sanela Unfirer, Dijana Kibel and
Aleksandar Kibel

Additional information is available at the end of the chapter

http://dx.doi.org/10.5772/intechopen.76569

Abstract

The mechanisms by which HBO exerts its potentially beneficial effects are not completely clear. Interactions of mechanisms affecting endothelial dysfunction, NO synthesis, EETs and HETE formation, CYP expression changes, oxidative stress and antioxidant defense system changes, and multiple effects on inflammation take place that might be considered as mediating factors for the observed positive (or negative) clinical effects in diabetes mellitus (for instance in chronic diabetic wounds). Studies on vasculature in diabetic animal models can provide us with more information that can help us understand its effects on blood vessel function. This chapter discusses the most relevant studies that have assessed the potential mechanisms of HBO-induced vascular functional changes in diabetic animal models.

Keywords: hyperbaric oxygen, diabetes mellitus, endothelial dysfunction, cytochrome P450, nitric oxide, arachidonic acid metabolites

1. Introduction

Hyperbaric oxygen (HBO) therapy presents medical and experimental administration of 100% oxygen (O_2) at pressures above 1 atm [1, 2]. HBO is widely used for the treatment of various clinical diseases, but numerous studies indicate its benefit in conditions of vascular pathology [2]. The exact mechanisms that are involved in the actions of therapy with HBO_2 are largely unknown, although its effects have been documented clinically and in experimental models [2,3]. Investigations focusing on physiological effects of hyperbaric oxygen on vascular function still do not provide a clear mechanism of its action. They focus on endothelial function and dysfunction, as well as HBO-induced changes in concentrations and actions of physiological mediators of vascular function, such as nitric oxide (NO), acetylcholine, metabolites of arachidonic acids, and others. Some works also suggest that HBO might cause changes in conducted vasomotor responses and in that way influences vascular sensitivity and reactivity to vasodilators and vasoconstrictors [4].

2. Endothelial function and dysfunction

Endothelial cells are responsible for vascular tone, supply the thromboresistance, and determine the extent to which the vasculature is permeable to cells and molecules through the synthesis and release of a wide variety of substances [5]. The pathogenetic concept of micro- and macroangiopathy, which are well-known vascular complications of diabetes mellitus (DM) [6], is based on an endothelial lesion that is a result of parameters specific for diabetes, which damage the endothelium [6]. Although basal tone and myogenic reactivity are intrinsic to vascular smooth muscle, the ambient level of tone is modulated by various vasoconstricting and vasodilating mediators released by the endothelium. It is generally accepted that long-term diabetes is associated with endothelial dysfunction and reduced endothelium-dependent vasodilation [7, 8]. The main endothelium-dependent vasodilatory mediator is NO, but various metabolites of arachidonic acid such as prostaglandins, epoxyeicosatrienoic acids (EETs), and hydroxyeicosatetraenoic acids (HETEs) also contribute to vascular responses to different stimuli [9, 10] and may be essential for vascular response in various physiologic and pathological conditions such as diabetes mellitus [11–13].

Hyperbaric oxygen therapy affects the function and structure of cerebral resistant arteries, which is impaired in DM and will have beneficiary effect on vascular function by modulating mechanisms of vascular responses to various dilator and constrictor agonists, leading to restored vascular reactivity. It has been demonstrated that hyperglycemia, acute or chronic, may cause several changes in vascular function, including a decrease in endothelium-dependent vasodilation and an increase in contractile response of vascular smooth muscle [14]. Impaired endothelium-dependent relaxation has been shown in various vascular beds of different animal models [15]. The mechanisms associated with these observations may include changes in synthesis, release, and degradation of various factors that are produced by endothelium. The most notable characteristic of endothelium dysfunction in DM is the vascular NO reduction. Various multiple mechanisms are involved in this effect, but it seems that increased level of oxidative stress is the first alteration that triggers several others. Furthermore, the vascular smooth muscle sensitivity may be reduced, which certifies the vascular studies in human and animal models of DM that showed reduced sensitivity of vascular smooth muscle to NO donors [16].

On the other side, endothelial dysfunction may also be related to the release of vasoconstrictor factors. In vessels of diabetics, there is an increase in endothelium-dependent vasoconstrictor mechanisms, mostly mediated by prostanoids, which play an important role in endothelium dysfunction. TxA2 plays a role in the reduced endothelium response in type 1 DM, but it may also be involved in the enhanced contractile response to vasoconstrictor stimuli [17]. Furthermore, hyperglycemia increases the COX-2 expression, causing enhanced release of vasoconstrictor and prostanoids [18]. Hyperglycemia not only modifies the profile of prostanoids, leading to alteration of vasomotor tone, but also increases the release of arachidonic acid by vascular cells [19].

An increasing number of evidence proposes that HBO induces neuronal nitric oxide (NO) synthase (NOS) activity, while the influence on endothelial NOS (eNOS) activity and vascular NO bioavailability remains unclear [20]. Thom et al. reported that NO bioavailability in rat and mouse cerebral cortex was increased during HBO exposure, and cerebral NO production was enlarged much more in knockout mice lacking genes for eNOS than in those lacking genes for nNOS [21]. Studies on conscious rats with inhibition of NOS were used to assess the dynamics of cerebral blood flow during hyperbaric oxygenation and had shown that hyperbaric oxygen changes cerebral blood flow and modulates oxygen neurotoxicity via eNOS and nNOS [22]. eNOS- and nNOS-deficient mice were used to study the contributive roles of the NOS isoforms in mediating changes in cerebral vascular tone in response to hyperoxia, and results demonstrate that under HBO, eNOS-derived NO is responsible for the early vasoconstriction, whereas late HBO-induced vasodilation depends upon both eNOS and nNOS [23].

3. Influence on arachidonic acid metabolites and the renin-angiotensin system

HBO should be viewed as a factor for increased availability of oxygen as an active molecule in changing vascular function. HBO, CYP450 activity alternations, and arachidonic acid (AA) metabolism are connected in many different pathways. Besides vascular reactivity changes due to epoxidation reactions, Hjelde et al. showed that anti-inflammatory effect of HBO is mediated by reducing expression of cyclooxygenase-2 and reducing the number of intercellular adhesion molecules and therefore reducing adhesion and infiltration of leucocytes [24].

In various aspects of metabolic diseases, evidence from different studies suggests a role for enzymes involved in arachidonic acid (AA) metabolism, including cytochrome P450 (CYP) epoxygenases and soluble epoxide hydrolase (sEH), and their eicosanoid metabolites (epoxyeicosatrienoic acids (EETs)) [25–27]. EETs have been shown to exert beneficial effects on diabetes-related endothelial dysfunction, enhanced cardio protection, and alleviation of diabetic nephropathy. In contrast, CYP4A proteins were upregulated in the livers of mice with genetically induced and diet-induced diabetes [28].

Arachidonic acid in endothelial cell can be metabolized in three different pathways: CYP450 enzymes (omega-hydroxylase and epoxygenase), cyclooxygenase and lipoxygenase, and non-enzymatic degradation of arachidonic acid in the presence of free radicals to isoprostane [29]. Epoxygenase is a cytochrome P450 family of enzymes (primarily CYP2C and CYP2J families), which in the endothelial cell produces 4 epoxyeicosatrienoic acid (EETs) isomers (5,6-EET, 8,9-EET, 11,12-EET, and 14,15-EET), of which 14,15-EETs and 11,12-EETs are the most active metabolites [30]. In most cell types and organs, EETs can be present as dihydroxyeicosatrienoic acids (DHETs) [31], which are more stable and less bioactive than EETs. DHETs are produced by sEH hydrolysis of EETs [32]. There is no evidence of EET production in a smooth muscle cell. In a smooth muscle cell, cytochrome P450 ω-hydroxylase promotes the production of

20-hydroxy-eicosatrinoic acid (20-HETE), which is a vasoconstrictor. Cyclooxygenase (COX) is an enzyme existing in two isoformes, COX-1 and COX-2, involved in the synthesis of prostanoid from arachidonic acid (AA). The resulting prostanoids act in contradiction, causing vasodilation (prostaglandin D2, prostaglandin E2, and prostacyclin I2) and vasoconstriction (prostaglandin F2α and thromboxane A2). Hypoxia activates the COX pathway, where mostly prostacyclin, PGI2, is generated. It diffuses into the smooth muscle cell in which it activates the enzyme adenylate cyclase and increases the amount of cyclic adenosine monophosphate (cAMP). cAMP promotes the opening of several types of potassium channels, resulting in hyperpolarization of the smooth muscle membrane with consequent vasodilation [33]. Lipoxygenase is an enzyme that from AA generates 12- and 15-hydroxy eicosatrienoic acids (HETEs) as the major active metabolites in the endothelial cell [29, 34].

Streptozocin-induced diabetes in rats (a model for type 1 diabetes mellitus) reduces the levels of protective EETs, and the reduced EET levels lead to exacerbation of stroke [35]. Tsai et al. showed impaired endothelium-dependent vasodilation of coronary arterioles caused by reduced CYP activity and EET production due to increased glucose-induced superoxide levels in coronary endothelial cells [36]. EETs might constitute a key link between insulin resistance and endothelial dysfunction [37]. Endothelial dysfunction in diabetes could also be related to the release of vasoconstrictor mediators, e.g., increased production of 20-HETE leading to activation of ROS through an NAD(P)H-dependent pathway. Diabetes alters CYP expression and 20-HETE formation, leading to upregulation of CYP4A isoforms and to elevated levels of 20-HETE [37]. Li et al. also suggested contribution of 20-HETE to endothelial dysfunction in diabetes and other insulin-resistant conditions showing the attenuation of diabetes-induced vascular dysfunction by using the 20-HETE inhibitor HET0016 [38]. Insulin-stimulated vasodilation mediated by the IRS-1/PI3K/AKT/eNOS pathway can be impaired by 20-HETE [39]. Issan et al. associated dysfunction of circulating endothelial progenitor cells and angiogenic capacity with increased levels of CYP-derived 20-HETE in diabetic patients with cardiac ischemia [39]. P450 4A metabolite 20-HETE by vascular tissue is directly dependent on the concentration of oxygen within the normal physiological range of blood and tissue PO_2 [40]. It is known that various arachidonic acid metabolites (prostaglandins, EETs, HETEs) and NO are of utmost importance in the mediation of vascular reactions to vasodilators and vasoconstrictors [41–46], including hypoxia and hyperoxia stimuli [46]. In conditions of reduced blood flow, the use of HBO can significantly increase tissue oxygenation. Although all P450 enzymes require molecular oxygen, the majority of them (such as those found in the liver) require only very low PO_2 levels for normal activity. Results from our previous study suggest that hyperbaric oxygen increases vascular sensitivity to EETs, instead of significantly increasing EET synthesis [3]. Our studies also show that HBO is a highly effective treatment for stroke even in the presence of long-term untreated diabetes, by inhibition of 20-HETE production [47]. Unfirer et al.'s study showed changes in the dilatation mechanisms in diabetic rats under the influence of hyperbaric oxygenation. It has been shown that hyperbaric oxygenation causes activation of the CYP450 epoxygenase pathway and increased EET production in diabetic animals exposed to HBO [13]. Furthermore, Kibel et al. showed a changed relaxation response to ANG-(1–7) influenced by HBO in healthy and diabetic animals, where they also linked to a changed mechanism and improved relaxation after HBO with CYP450 activation and EET synthesis [3, 11]. HBO was shown to increase relaxation responses to ANG-(1–7) in rat aortic rings of diabetic animals, and this effect was eliminated with the addition of an EET synthesis inhibitor. There was no effect of HBO on ANGII reactivity of these aortic ring preparations nor was there a difference in serum concentrations of ANG-(1–7) [3]. mRNA and protein expression of several CYP isoforms that are involved in EET synthesis were also shown to be upregulated in aortic samples of animals, where DM was caused by streptozocin [3].

Both HBO as a treatment and in vitro hyperbaric oxygenation have been shown to change reactivity of rat thoracic aortic ring preparations to certain compounds [20, 48]. It is well known that changes in oxygen availability are crucial in the control of vascular tone, leading to changes in production of, or vessel sensitivity to, vasoconstrictor and vasodilator metabolites of arachidonic acid and nitric oxide (NO) [40, 49, 50]. The production of EETs is known to be reduced with a decrease in PO_2 [42]. EETs have been recognized to induce vasorelaxation and enhance K^+ current in smooth muscle cells, in addition to others (including pro-angiogenic, anti-inflammatory, and pro-fibrinolytic effects) [51–54].

CYP P450 3A13 was found to be involved in oxygen sensing, mediating ductus arteriosus constriction to oxygen, together with endothelin-1 [55]. Considering this, along with the interaction of arachidonic acid pathways with nitric oxide pathways in oxygen sensitivity [49], regional differences of arachidonic acid metabolite roles, and various conflicting evidence [49], it is clear that role of CYP450 enzymes in oxygen homeostasis is very complex and may be significant factor mediating the responses to HBO.

4. Changes in acetylcholine pathways

In the literature, there are a lot of studies on animal models of diabetes mellitus that confirmed impaired mechanisms of vasodilation and vasoconstriction. Streptozotocin-induced diabetes mellitus in rats demonstrates attenuated vasodilation response to acetylcholine [56, 57]. Experiments on healthy mouse coronary arteries demonstrate that vasodilation to acetylcholine is accomplished 50% by NO and 50% by EDHF. In spontaneously diabetic mouse type II (db/db), that ratio is 81% to production of EDHF [12].

Unfirer et al. [13] first investigated mechanisms of vasorelaxation in diabetic animal models after HBO exposure. Thoracic aortal rings from SD rats were used to evaluate vasorelaxation responses to acetylcholine after preconstruction with noradrenalin. With NG-nitro-L-arginine methyl ester (L-NAME)-(NOS inhibitor), indomethacin-(COX inhibitor), and N-(methylsulfonyl)-2-(2-propynyloxy)-benzenehexanamide (MS-PPOH)-(CYP 450-epoxygenase inhibitor), they investigated which pathway is involved in enhanced vasorelaxation responses in diabetic and healthy rats after HBO exposure. HBO exposure protocol was performed in therapeutic range [58]. DM duration of 6 weeks did not change vasorelaxation response in diabetic group, and after application of inhibitors, results showed that the NO pathway is dominant in macrocirculation. In the diabetic and healthy groups, after HBO exposure, there was partial inhibition of vasorelaxation after NOS inhibition, which indicates that other pathways were included in vasorelaxation mechanisms. MS-PPOH partially blocked vasorelaxation in both HBO groups, which indicates that HBO changes vasorelaxation mechanisms to alternative pathways—enhanced production or sensitivity to EETs. Indomethacin did not inhibit vasorelaxation in any group, so COX pathway did not have influence. These findings were verified with upregulation of eNOS and COX-1 enzymes in the diabetic HBO group and higher protein expression of CYP450-4A1/A2/A3 in both HBO groups when compared with their respective controls. Also in this study, there was not oxidative stress caused by HBO because thiobarbituric acid-reactive substances (TBARSs) were elevated in DM group but were normal in the healthy HBO group. This difference between studies is probably a result of different experimental protocols (intermittent hyperbaric oxygenation—2 hours, 4 days at 2.0 atm abs vs. 90 minutes, 7 days at 2.4 atm abs in Matsunami study [59]).

Same authors investigate HBO effect on microcirculation (middle cerebral arteries) in diabetic animal model, 6-week duration of DM. Preliminary results shown impaired vasodilation response in diabetic rats and restored vasodilation after HBO exposure. Using inhibitors such as indomethacin (COX), NG-monomethyl-L-arginine (L-NMMA) (NOS), and clotrimazole (nonselective CYP 450 inhibitor), they notice shift in vasodilation mechanisms from mainly NO pathway toward two other pathways COX/CYP 450 because in both HBO groups, L-NMMA did not blocked vasodilation to acetylcholine. Further investigation is necessary [60].

In normal condition, vasodilation response to hypoxia is made by activating cyclooxygenase (COX) and production of prostacyclin (PGI2) [61]. There is evidence that CYP 450-epoxigenase enzyme in minor part causes vasodilation in healthy vessels [62]. Experiments on middle cerebral arteries (MCAs) of 6 weeks diabetic rats that underwent HBO exposure were used to evaluate the effect of HBO in acute hypoxia. They used COX inhibitor indomethacin and selective CYP 450 epoxygenase inhibitor MS-PPOH. COX inhibition partially preserved vasodilation in HBO groups, and eliminated vasodilation in response to hypoxia in the presence of MS-PPOH in both HBO groups suggests that HBO activates CYP450-epoxigenase in MCAs of healthy and DM rats and shifts vasodilation mechanisms in response to acute hypoxia [63].

5. Effects on oxidative stress [reactive oxygen species (ROS)]

Life on Earth is impossible without oxygen that is in our atmosphere, which consists of 21% oxygen. Paradoxically, oxygen can also potentially be very toxic for organisms that use it. Free radical formation occurs continuously in cells as a consequence of both enzymatic and nonenzymatic reactions [64]. The main compartments of these kinds of reactions in cells are mitochondria. Mediated by nicotinamide adenine dinucleotide phosphate (NADPH) oxidase, mitochondria are the site of significant reactive oxygen species (ROS) production [65]. The term "ROS" is generally used to describe reactive molecules containing oxygen. Such molecules have many common and similar characteristics; they also exhibit very different features, resulting in potentially beneficial or even toxic effects [66]. On the other hand, the term reactive oxygen species (ROS) can be defined as highly reactive oxygen-centered chemical species containing one or two unpaired electrons, where an unpaired electron is one that exists in an atomic or molecular orbital alone. The unpaired electron containing chemical species can also be called "free radicals." Furthermore, the term "ROS" can also be used as a "collective term" to include both radicals and nonradicals, the latter being devoid of unpaired electrons. So, ROS is classified into two categories: (1) oxygen-centered radicals and (2) oxygen-centered nonradicals. Oxygen-centered radicals include superoxide anion ($^{\cdot}O^{2-}$), hydroxyl radical ($^{\cdot}OH$), alkoxyl radical ($RO^{\cdot}$), and peroxyl radical ($ROO^{\cdot}$). Oxygen-centered nonradicals are

http://dx.doi.org/10.5772/intechopen.76569

hydrogen peroxide (H_2O_2), singlet oxygen (O_2, high-energy form of oxygen), and hypochlorous acids (HOCl) [67]. Sometimes when ROSs break the upper concentration limit of cellular antioxidant defense system capacity, based on high ROS intracellular concentration or low cellular antioxidant defense system, oxidative stress will show up and manifest with nucleic acids, proteins, and lipids damage, leading to carcinogenesis, neurodegenerative disorders, atherosclerosis, diabetes, and aging [68]. Under normal physiological conditions, ROS and the peroxidized molecules are neutralized by a powerful antioxidant system involving superoxide dismutases, catalases, glutathione S-transferases, and thioredoxins [69].

In diabetes and hyperglycemia in general, NADPH oxidase represents the principal source of ROS production in different organs [67]. The most acceptable thesis is that oxidative stress, as a main result of HBO, is a major trigger of most of its effects, but the exact mechanisms are not completely clear. It could be confusing to understand different consequences of HBO depending on protocol type that was used. For example, the duration of exposure, the used oxygen pressure, the subject species, and the underlying disease are factors that may play a role in changes of blood pressure levels [70], and changes of specific oxidative parameters depend on lapsed time after exposure or on the number of repeated exposures (analyzing rat lung tissue) [71, 72]. Although increased superoxide dismutase and glutathione peroxidase activity and increased thiobarbituric acid-reactive substance levels are documented, after some hyperbaric protocols, there is no change in aforementioned enzyme concentrations in red blood cells. On the other hand, a significant induction of heat shock protein HSP70 in lymphocytes after even a single HBO_2 treatment was noted—this might be due to activation of compensatory mechanisms by HBO_2 [70]. After hyperbaric treatment with high oxygen concentration, an increased ROS production is noticed, but paradoxically, HBO induces an antioxidant environment in plasma by increasing the plasma catalase activity. Different studies have documented increases in the total plasma antioxidant capacity determined after a session with HBO [73]. The therapeutic use of HBO can give positive results by activation of ROS resulting in increased perfusion, reduced edema, decreased inflammatory cytokines, increased fibroblast proliferation, increased collagen production, and angiogenesis promotion. Finally, increase of ROS may improve the regulation of antioxidant enzyme activity of tissues [74].

6. Inflammation

Pathological effects of DM on the vascular wall include enhanced ROS production and endothelial activation leading to inflammation, atherogenesis, and vascular dysfunction, which further results in clinical impairment of the micro- and macrocirculation. Interestingly, positive therapeutic effects of HBO_2, such as antioxidative and anti-inflammatory effects, have been attributed to the enhanced ROS production induced by the HBO_2 treatment [1].

Numerous studies on experimental DM animal models revealed ongoing vascular inflammation under diabetic/hyperglycemic conditions, characterized by (a) increased proinflammatory cytokine levels, including interleukin-6 (IL-6) and tumor necrosis factor alpha (TNF-α); (b) endothelial activation followed by increased expression of vascular cellular adhesion molecule-1 (VCAM-1);

and (c) increased leukocyte homing to the vessels and tissues induced by excessive secretion of chemokines like monocyte chemoattractant protein (MCP-1) [75–77]. In addition to that, same noxa that lead to inflammation also precipitate development of vascular dysfunction, marked by substantial decrease in NO bioavailability, which is discussed in more detail elsewhere in this chapter [78]. Studies on diabetic (db/db) and control (db/+) mice have shown that DM prolongs the inflammatory response to a bacterial stimulus through cytokine dysregulation, particularly the TNF-α [79]. Similar results were also obtained from experiments using type 1 DM animal model (mice receiving multiple low-dose streptozotocin treatments), suggesting that the observed proinflammatory status of diabetic mice is predominately linked to hyperglycemia rather than pathomechanism involved in the development of a specific type of DM [80]. Additionally, impaired function of macrophages, including reduced efferocytosis and anti-inflammatory cytokine expression, has been attributed to the prolonged and ineffective resolution of inflammation in the wounds of diabetic mice, which is a leading complication in diabetic humans [81]. This was further confirmed by intravital microscopy that allowed researchers to real-time follow-up leukocytes in live diabetic and healthy control mice, which was followed by leukocyte isolation and functional tests that all together revealed enhanced recruitment but defective function of leukocytes during the inflammation in mouse models of type 1 and type 2 DM resulting in defective bacterial clearance [82]. Studies have also shown that hyperglycemia changes the intrinsic TCR-induced naïve T activation to increased T cell responsiveness in diabetes [83]. In the kidneys, the observed proinflammatory condition in DM animals has been linked to oxidative stress-induced JNK activation [84]. It has also been shown that diabetic condition facilitates binding of monocytes to vascular smooth muscle cells and their subsequent differentiation through induction of key chemokines in the vasculature, which can lead to enhanced atherogenesis [85]. In addition, endothelial cells (EC) express pattern-recognition receptors including Toll-like receptors (TLR) that have a central role in recognizing pathogens and damage signals and initiating immune responses [86]. It seems that in the vessels of diabetic animals/individuals, increased oxidative stress, free fatty acids, and hyperglycemia are directly involved in the pathogenesis of vascular inflammation via several cellular mechanisms, including TLR-mediated activation of protein kinase C (PKC) and NF-κB pathways resulting in increased expression of the proinflammatory molecules such as IL-6 and TNF-α. In turn, secretion of cytokines IL-1 and TNF-α increases NF-κB activity and production of cellular adhesion molecules by endothelial cells, further aggravating the inflammation [87].

Some of the beneficial anti-inflammatory effects of HBO include reduced proinflammatory cytokine expression, suppressed development of T helper cells, shrinking of spleen and lymph nodes, decreased responses to antigens, recruitment and differentiation of circulating stem cells, and reduced frequencies of circulating leukocytes [88, 89]. However, these effects were mainly observed in studies exploring experimental animal models of colitis, while in the particular case of DM, data on the effects of HBO on the vascular inflammation are scarce. This is in contrast to our knowledge about the effects of the HBO on the wound-healing mechanisms that have been subjects of intensive investigations for many years, which lead to profound understanding of the clinically observed positive effects of HBO [90].

Beneficial effects of HBO on the wound-healing processes include facilitation of the neovascularization through enhanced regional angiogenic stimuli and increased recruitment and differentiation of circulating stem cells from the bone marrow [1]. Under ischemic and hyperglycemic conditions, HBO further promotes wound repair by increasing tissue perfusion and collagen deposition [91]. A study on an experimental wound model revealed increased synthesis of vascular endothelial growth factor (VEGF) in damaged tissue during HBO_2, which is the most specific growth factor for neovascularization [92]. It is controversial that HBO_2-induced oxidative stress leads to hypoxia-inducible factor (HIF)-1 and 2 mediated transcriptions of many genes involved with neovascularization, including stromal-derived factor-1 (SDF-1) and its counterpart ligand, CXCR4, as well as VEGF [1]. These effects could be especially beneficial for DM individuals whose stem cell mobilization is compromised by impaired NOS activity in the bone marrow [1].

It has been shown that HBO inhibits ischemia reperfusion induced β2-integrin-dependent adhesion of neutrophils to the endothelium by blocking CD18 surface polarization and through S-nitrosation of β2-integrin, with no effect on the cell-surface expression of β2-integrins [93]. Studies on monocyte-macrophages retrieved from healthy humans and animals exposed to HBO in vivo or cells exposed to HBO under in vitro condition revealed lower stimulus-induced proinflammatory cytokine production upon exposure to HBO_2 [1, 94].

Studies on ApoE KO mice that exhibit accelerated atherosclerosis and related complications showed that HBO_2 reduces the circulating levels of antibodies to $_{MDA}$LDL and dampens delayed hypersensitivity response to oxLDL challenge. The same studies demonstrated significant reduction in the production of proinflammatory cytokines, along with marked increase in the constitutive production of the anti-inflammatory cytokine IL-10 in splenocytes stimulated by LPS [95]. This effect was independent of antigen specificity, as indicated by polyclonal activation of T cells.

7. The role of HBO in stroke

Approximately 25% of all stroke patients have DM and 40% have hyperglycemia, which is associated with worse neurologic outcome as well as higher risk of recurrence of stroke [96, 97]. Diabetic patients, compared to nondiabetics, are known to be more sensitive to cerebral ischemia. Thus, the same duration of ischemia results in more severe neurologic deficits and larger brain infarcts in diabetic patients. Female patients with DM have 4.8-fold higher risk for developing ischemic stroke than the general population (compared to 3.7-fold for men) and more often suffer fatal strokes (standardized mortality ratios of 3.1 for males and 4.4 for females) [98–100]. The outcome is frequently lethal, regardless of any therapy undertaken, including recombinant tissue plasminogen activator (rtPA) and mechanical thrombectomy. Possible underlying causes are chronic hyperglycemia, which leads to free oxygen radicals and cytokines production and increases ischemic brain cells predisposition to apoptosis [101]. In addition, the intimal artery thickening and arteriolar occlusion occur in diabetes, contributing by impaired vascular function to inadequate tissue perfusion. Moreover, DM is, in some cases, such as treatment of recurrent stroke with thrombolysis, one of the exclusion criteria [102].

A total of 90–95% diabetic patients are type 2 DM of noninsulin dependence and 5–10% are type 1 DM of insulin dependence. Type 2 DM patients have asymptomatic period of hyperglycemia for about 4–7 years that leads to most important problems—chronic complications of diabetes, leading to disability and premature death [103]. First diabetic complications are associated with microangiopathy of retina, kidney, and peripheral neuropathy and next with macroangiopathy causing myocardial infarction, stroke, hypertension, and peripheral artery lesion. Patients with DM have progressive cerebrovascular atherosclerosis and increased cerebral vascular reaction to vascular constrictors, a deregulated reaction to vascular dilators and damaged automatic regulation of brain-blood stream. Damaged endothelium and vascular motor function of small arteries can lead to hypoperfusion of certain areas of the brain in diabetic patients.

The principles of HBO are based on physical laws and mechanisms of oxygen transport in human body. At sea level (1 ATA), almost all hemoglobin is saturated with oxygen, and HBO can increase its saturation only slightly. However, HBO increases the amount of oxygen dissolved in plasma from 0.3 to 5.6% at 2.5 ATA, and due to this mechanism, it increases tissue oxygenation even in areas where erythrocytes cannot pass [104]. Due to oxygen pressure gradient, HBO promotes diffusion of oxygen to longer distances in ischemic region. HBO_2 raises oxygenation of ischemic penumbra by 20% and improves mitochondrial function [105, 106]. Single or multiple exposures to HBO create environment of intermittent relative hypoxia that can not only prepare tissue for longer hypoxia but also save tissue until other salvation strategies (such as thrombolysis, mechanical thrombectomy, stenting, and endarterectomy) take effect [47, 107]. Not only oxygen in ischemic core and penumbra itself plays a vital role in surviving tissues; HBO also influences on many different pathophysiological mechanisms. HBO improves oxygen delivery to ischemic brain tissue due to the higher arterial blood-brain oxygen gradient.

In animal models, it stabilizes blood-brain barrier (BBB) and therefore reduces brain edema formation. It improves brain microcirculation and brain metabolism, creating sufficient energy and ion homeostasis needed for survival of cells until reperfusion or collateral circulation creation. Some concern was about vasoconstriction of arteries under HBO. This can be applied to normal, but not ischemic vessels, where secondary vasodilatation is salvation mechanism and vasoconstriction does not appear. HBO actually improves microcirculation in ischemic areas [108, 109]. HBO reduces poststroke inflammation by various mechanisms, reduces the number of brain cells undergoing apoptotic pathways and necrotic death, and if applied early, it can reduce ischemia-reperfusion injury and reduce oxidative stress. These combined effects reduce brain edema and modulate cerebral vascular flow resulting in reduced intracranial pressure. Longer effects of HBO include promotion of angiogenesis and neurogenesis in ischemic tissues with positive effect on neurorehabilitation. In numerous animal experimental models, HBO was effective in reducing brain infarction after stroke. However, few human studies were so successful.

HBO has been used in humans in many different stroke types (hemorrhagic, ischemic, large and small artery stroke, global ischemia, etc.) using different pressures, protocols of application (single or multiple) and in different poststroke time windows. Due to these inconsistent standards, some studies showed lack of effect and other benefits. Another point of concern is that only the small number of these studies were well-designed randomized controlled trials and that their limitations include the small number of patients, which means that precise conclusions cannot be drawn. Some cautious conclusions could be suggested. HBO is so far the only effective early treatment of air embolism (mostly after surgery). HBO early after stroke improves recovery after stroke, but this effect progressively decreases if treatment is applied later. The most significant results are achieved in first 3 hours after stroke (similar to thrombolysis and other revascularization trials). Time window for HBO is 3–6 hours in acute ischemic stroke. The question of later and repetitive administration of HBO shows some promising results; however, they are still based on a few clinical cases and lack scientific proof and larger number of cases. Multiple repetitive HBO has positive effect on cognitive recovery after stroke and metabolism of temporal lobe. In one clinical trial, HBO combined with antidepressants showed better results than any of these therapies alone. HBO reduces cerebrovascular vasospasm and secondary brain infarctions after aneurismal subarachnoid hemorrhage (SAH). In intracerebral hemorrhage patients, HBO also provided improvement if started early, and the patient is stable [110].

When one thinks about treating acute stroke in diabetic patients with HBO, a few still unanswered questions arise, mostly due to the paucity of experiments in these settings. There are a few experiments conducted in animal models, but they vary in criteria for its use. In humans, we can rely only on a small number of cases with very diverse inclusion criteria and different results. Therefore, we can only draw some direct and more indirect conclusions about it from experiments on nondiabetic stroke experiments.

There is a question of optimal model of animal stroke in diabetic animals. The most commonly used experimental model of stroke in rats is a model of middle cerebral artery occlusion (MCAO) by intra-luminal suture. There are variations of this model in terms of use of permanent or transitory MCA occlusion-induced ischemia. The duration of occlusion varies in models from permanent MCAO to transitory MCAO (t-MCAO) of 180, 120, 105, or 60 minutes [111]. Taking into account the observed differences in clinical presentation of diabetic vs. nondiabetic patients with stroke, there are few issues that variations in experimental approach to stroke study are brought to light. For example, in diabetic rat stroke models, the same duration of MCAO as in nondiabetic rat models is used.

The usual duration of t-MCAO used in non-diabetic rats was 60-120 minute [112]. In diabetic rats the same duration of t-MCAO produced massive stroke with malignant brain edema, devastating neurological deficits (such as inability to move, eat and drink) that become worse over time, leading to unconsciousness and death of animals within the first 24 hours (mostly due to massive edema and a rise in intracranial pressure). If ischemia lasts too long, laser Doppler flowmetry (LDF) finds lesser than expected reperfusional values. This brain vascular sign could be a marker of point of no return in stroke treatment [111]. Therefore (to develop the adequate diabetic female rat model, using transitory middle cerebral artery occlusion (t-MCAO) that would produce treatable stroke conditions in rats with diabetes), one has to significantly shorten the duration of t-MCAO to avoid already-irreversible brain infarct with brain vascular derangement. One study suggests that 30-minute t-MCAO could be a more appropriate stroke model than the usual 60-120 minute t-MCAO models, consistently producing medium-sized stroke, which affects 30–50% of ischemic hemisphere [111] (865443). Similarly, patients with the most severe strokes of the whole MCA territory and high National Institute of Health Stroke Score (NIHSS) not only are poor candidates for treatment with thrombolysis and mostly die due to brain edema and complications of dysphagia and immobility, but also have higher risk of secondary hemorrhage.

In conclusion, it is questionable to compare results of artery occlusion for rats with and without diabetes, even if the duration of t-MCAO is equal.

The only effective pharmacological therapy of acute ischemic stroke in humans is thrombolysis with recombinant tissue plasminogen activator, but DM is sometimes an exclusion criterion in recurrent stroke treatment. The time window for the therapy is narrow, and no other pharmacological agents have demonstrated efficacy in improving outcomes after ischemic stroke [1–4, 100, 102]. Thus, the searches for alternative approaches are welcomed. HBO [113] improves oxygen delivery and postischemic metabolism, restores ion pump function, and allows time for collateral circulation to develop [107]. In normal tissue, it causes vasoconstriction, but in ischemic brain tissue, it increases microvascular flow and improves oxygen dissolution and transport [109]. Time window for HBO application may be up to 6 hours [108], which is longer than the time window for thrombolytic therapy. HBO raises oxygenation of ischemic penumbra by 20% and improves mitochondrial function [107, 108]. It has anti-inflammatory effect by reducing expression of cyclooxygenase-2 and reduces the number of intercellular adhesion molecules and therefore reduces adhesion and infiltration of leukocytes [24]. However, guidelines do not recommend HBO treatment for acute ischemic stroke due to somewhat inconclusive data [102]. Some data imply that the intervention may be harmful causing middle ear trauma, epileptic seizures, and claustrophobia, while others found no firm evidence that HBO improves clinical outcomes for acute stroke. However, the main disadvantage of these trials used in meta-analysis was delay from stroke onset to initiation of HBO and the need for care delivery in a specialized chamber [114].

To conclude, HBO is currently not recommended for patients with acute ischemic stroke outside of clinical trials (except caused by air embolism).

On the other hand, some preclinical experiments suggest that if administered shortly after the stroke, HBO is highly effective treatment of stroke in diabetic female rats, even in the presence of long-term untreated DM [109]. Experiments that did not show effectiveness of HBO were possibly unsuccessful due to the unrecognizing the vulnerability of neurons. They used prolonged ischemia and applied HBO treatment too late after stroke.

8. Conclusion

The mechanisms by which HBO exerts its potentially beneficial effects are not completely clear. They cannot be simply explained as a consequence of supplementation of the oxygen deficit in certain conditions where oxygen is lacking, but it was demonstrated that HBO affects signaling cascades in cells and has multiple interacting complex mechanisms that might contribute to functional changes of blood vessels. Interactions of mechanisms affecting endothelial dysfunction, NO synthesis, EETs formation, CYP expression changes, oxidative stress and antioxidant defense system changes, and multiple effects on inflammation take place that might be considered as mediating factors for the observed positive (or negative) clinical effects in diabetes mellitus (for instance in chronic diabetic wounds). Studies on vasculature in diabetic animal models can provide us with more information that can help us understand its effects on blood vessel function, and **Table 1** summarizes the most relevant mechanisms that have been described in this text regarding functional vascular changes in

Target group of mechanisms or single mechanism	Effect	References
Endothelial dysfunction	↑ NO bioavailability	[20–23]
Arachidonic acid metabolites	↑ EETs synthesis, CYP epoxygenase expression, vascular sensitivity to EETs (?) ↓ 20-HETE	[2, 3, 11, 13, 47]
Oxidative stress	↑ ROS ↑ Antioxidant defense systems (?)	[2, 70–74]
Inflammation	↓ Proinflammatory mediators ↑Angiogenic mediators	[1, 2, 90–94]
Renin-angiotensin system	↑ Vascular reactivity to ANG-(1–7)	[2, 3, 11]
Physical effects	↑ Dissolved oxygen in plasma and tissues	[104–106]

Table 1. Major potential mechanisms of HBO-induced vascular functional changes in diabetic animal models.

animal experimental models of diabetes. However, this represents only a part of the complete picture, and further studies are necessary to completely elucidate all the mechanisms involved in the effects of HBO on blood vessels.

Conflict of interest

The authors have no conflict of interest to declare.

Author details

Ivana Jukic[1], Mihael Mišir[1,2], Martina Mihalj[1], Zrinka Mihaljevic[1], Sanela Unfirer[1,3], Dijana Kibel[1,4] and Aleksandar Kibel[1,5]*

*Address all correspondence to: aleksandar_mf@yahoo.com

1 Department of Physiology and Immunology, Faculty of Medicine, University of Osijek, Osijek, Croatia

2 Neurological Clinic, Osijek University Hospital, Osijek, Croatia

3 Emergency Department, Osijek University Hospital, Osijek, Croatia

4 Department of Diagnostic and Interventional Radiology, Osijek University Hospital, Osijek, Croatia

5 Department for Heart and Vascular Diseases, Osijek University Hospital, Osijek, Croatia

References

[1] Thom SR. Oxidative stress is fundamental to hyperbaric oxygen therapy. Journal of Applied Physiology (1985). Mar 2009;**106**(3):988-995

[2] Drenjancevic I, Kibel A. Restoring vascular function with hyperbaric oxygen treatment: Recovery mechanisms. Journal of Vascular Research. 2014;**51**:1-13

[3] Kibel A, Novak S, Cosic A, Mihaljevic Z, Falck JR, Drenjancevic I. Hyperbaric oxygenation modulates vascular reactivity to angiotensin-(1-7) in diabetic rats: Potential role of epoxyeicosatrienoic acids. Diabetes & Vascular Disease Research. Jan 2015;**12**(1):33-45

[4] Drenjančević-Perić I, Gros M, Kibel A. Influence of hyperbaric oxygen on blood vessel reactivity: Concept of changes in conducted vasomotor response. Collegium Antropologicum. Jun 2009;**33**(2):681-685

[5] Sandoo A, van Zanten JJ, Metsios GS, Carroll D, Kitas GD. The endothelium and its role in regulating vascular tone. Open Cardiovascular Medicine Journal. Dec 23, 2010;**4**:302-312

[6] Gärtner V, Eigentler TK. Pathogenesis of diabetic macroand microangiopathy. Clinical Nephrology. 2008;**70**(1):1-9

[7] Fujii KD, Heistad D, Faraci FM. Effect of diabetes mellitus on flow-mediated and endothelium-dependent dilation of the rat basilar artery. Stroke. 1992;**23**:1494-1498

[8] Mayhan WG, Simmons LK, Sharpe GM. Mechanism of impaired responses of cerebral arterioles during diabetes mellitus. The American Journal of Physiology. 1991;**260**: H319-H326

[9] Armitage ME, Wingler K, Schmidt HH, La M. Translating the oxidative stress hypothesis into the clinic: NOX versus NOS. Journal of Molecular Medicine. 2009;**87**(11):1071-1076

[10] Vallance PJT, Webb DJ, eds. Chapter 12: The eicosanoids: Cyclooxygenase, lipoxygenase and epoxygenase pathways. In: Vascular Endothelium in Human Physiology and Pathophysiology. 2008. pp. 332-361

[11] Kibel A, Cavka A, Cosic A, Falck JR, Drenjancevic I. Effects of hyperbaric oxygenation on vascular reactivity to angiotensin II and angiotensin-[1-7] in rats. Undersea & Hyperbaric Medicine. 2012;**39**(6):1053-1066

[12] Park Y, Capobianco S, Gao X, Falck JR, Dellsperger KC, Zhang C. Role of EDHF in type 2 diabetes-induced endothelial dysfunction. American Journal of Physiology. Heart and Circulatory Physiology. 2008;**295**(5):H1982-H1988

[13] Unfirer S, Mihalj M, Novak S, Kibel A, Cavka A, Mijalevic Z, Gros M, Brizic I, Budimir D, Cosic A, Boban M, Drenjancevic I. Hyperbaric oxygenation affects the mechanisms of acetylcholine-induced relaxation in diabetic rats. Undersea & Hyperbaric Medicine. 2016 Nov-Dec;**43**(7):787-803

[14] Davel AP, Wenceslau CF, Akamine EH, Xavier FE, Couto GK, Oliveira HT, Rossoni LV. Endothelial dysfunction in cardiovascular and endocrine-metabolic diseases: An update. Brazilian Journal of Medical and Biological Research. 2011 Sep;**44**(9):920-932

[15] Pieper GM. Enhanced, unaltered and impaired nitric oxidemediated endothelium-dependent relaxation in experimental diabetes mellitus: Importance of disease duration. Diabetologia. 1999;**42**:204-213

[16] Chan NN, Vallance P, Colhoun HM. Endothelium-dependent and -independent vascular dysfunction in type 1 diabetes: Role of conventional risk factors, sex, and glycemic control. Arteriosclerosis, Thrombosis, and Vascular Biology. 2003;**23**:1048-1054

[17] Xavier FE, Davel AP, Rossoni LV, Vassallo DV. Time-dependent hyperreactivity to phenylephrine in aorta from untreated diabetic rats: Role of prostanoids and calcium mobilization. Vascular Pharmacology. 2003;**40**:67-76

[18] Bagi Z, Erdei N, Papp Z, Edes I, Koller A. Up-regulation of vascular cyclooxygenase-2 in diabetes mellitus. Pharmacological Reports. 2006;**58**(Suppl):52-56

[19] Tesfamariam B, Brown ML, Deykin D, Cohen RA. Elevated glucose promotes generation of endothelium-derived vasoconstrictor prostanoids in rabbit aorta. The Journal of Clinical Investigation. 1990;**85**:929-932

[20] Hink J, Thom SR, Simonsen U, Rubin I, Jansen E. Vascular reactivity and endothelial NOS activity in rat thoracic aorta during and after hyperbaric oxygen exposure. American Journal of Physiology. Heart and Circulatory Physiology. 2006 Oct;**291**(4):H1988-H1998

[21] Thom SR, Bhopale V, Fisher D, Manevich Y, Huang PL, Buerk DG. Stimulation of nitric oxide synthase in cerebral cortex due to elevated partial pressures of oxygen: An oxidative stress response. Journal of Neurobiology. 2002;**51**:85-100

[22] Moskvin AN, Zhilyaev SY, Sharapov OI, Platonova TF, Gutsaeva DR, Kostkin VB, Demchenko IT. Brain blood flow modulates the neurotoxic action of hyperbaric oxygen via neuronal and endothelial nitric oxide. Neuroscience and Behavioral Physiology. 2003;**33**(9):883-888

[23] Atochin DN, Demchenko IT, Astern J, Boso AE, Piantadosi CA, Huang PL. Contributions of endothelial and neuronal nitric oxide synthases to cerebrovascular responses to hyperoxia. Journal of Cerebral Blood Flow and Metabolism. 2003;**23**(10):1219-1226

[24] Hjelde A, Hjelstuen M, Haraldseth O, Martin D, Thom R, Brubakk O. Hyperbaric oxygen and neutrophil accumulation/tissue damage during permanent focal cerebral ischaemia in rats. European Journal of Applied Physiology. 2002;**86**:401-405

[25] Luria A, Bettaieb A, Xi Y, Shieh GJ, Liu HC, Inoue H, Tsai HJ, Imig JD, Haj FG, Hammock BD. Soluble epoxide hydrolase deficiency alters pancreatic islet size and improves glucose homeostasis in a model of insulin resistance. Proceedings of the National Academy of Sciences of the United States of America. 2011 May 31;**108**(22):9038-9043

[26] Xu X, Zhao CX, Wang L, Tu L, Fang X, Zheng C, Edin ML, Zeldin DC, Wang DW. Increased CYP2J3 expression reduces insulin resistance in fructose-treated rats and db/db mice. Diabetes. Apr 2010;**59**(4):997-1005

[27] Xu X, Li R, Chen G, Hoopes SL, Zeldin DC, Wang DW. The role of cytochrome P450 epoxygenases, soluble epoxide hydrolase, and epoxyeicosatrienoic acids in metabolic

diseases. Advances in Nutrition. Nov 2016;7(6):1122-1128. Published online: Nov 10, 2016. DOI: 10.3945/an.116.012245

[28] Park EC, Kim SI, Hong Y, Hwang JW, Cho GS, Cha HN, Han JK, Yun CH, Park SY, Jang IS, Lee ZW, Choi JS, Kim S, Kim GH. Inhibition of CYP4A reduces hepatic endoplasmic reticulum stress and features of diabetes in mice. Gastroenterology. Oct 2014;**147**(4):860-869

[29] Drenjančević I, Jukić I, Mihaljević Z, Ćosić A, Kibel A. The metabolites of arachidonic acid in microvascular function. In: Lenasi H, editor. Microcirculation Revisited – From Molecules to Clinical Practice. Rijeka: InTech: 2016. pp. 101-133

[30] Bellien J, Joannides R. Epoxyeicosatrienoic acid pathway in human health and diseases. Journal of Cardiovascular Pharmacology. Mar 2013;**61**(3):188-196

[31] Imig JD, Hammock BD. Soluble epoxide hydrolase as a therapeutic target for cardiovascular diseases. Nature Reviews. Drug Discovery. Oct 2009;**8**(10):794-805

[32] Capdevila J, Wang W. Role of cytochrome P450 epoxygenase in regulating renal membrane transport and hypertension. Current Opinion in Nephrology and Hypertension. 2013 Mar;**22**(2):163-169

[33] Félétou M, Huang Y, Vanhoutte PM. Endothelium-mediated control of vascular tone: COX-1 and COX-2 products. British Journal of Pharmacology. 2011;**164**:894-912

[34] Imig JD. Epoxides and soluble epoxide hydrolase in cardiovascular physiology. Physiological Reviews. 2012 January;**92**(1):101-130

[35] Jouihan SA, Zuloaga KL, Zhang W, Shangraw RE, Krasnow SM, Marks DL, et al. Role of soluble epoxide hydrolase in exacerbation of stroke by streptozotocin-induced type 1 diabetes mellitus. Journal of Cerebral Blood Flow & Metabolism. 2013;**33**:1650-1656

[36] Tsai SH, Hein TW, Kuo L, YangVC.High glucose impairs EDHF-mediated dilation of coronary arterioles via reduced cytochrome P450 activity. Microvascular Research. 2011;**82**(3):356-363

[37] Mustafa S, Sharma V, McNeill JH. Insulin resistance and endothelial dysfunction: Are epoxyeicosatrienoicacids the link? Experimental & Clinical Cardiology. 2009;**14**:e41-e50

[38] Li X, Zhao G, Ma B, Li R, Hong J, Liu S, Wang DW. 20-Hydroxyeicosatetraenoic acid impairs endothelial insulin signaling by inducing phosphorylation of the insulin receptor substrate-1 at Ser616. PLoS One. 2014;**9**(4):e95841

[39] Issan Y, Hochhauser E, Guo A, Gotlinger KH, Kornowski R, Leshem-Lev D, Lev E, Porat E, Snir E, Thompson CI, Abraham NG, Laniado-Schwartzman M. Elevated level of proinflammatory eicosanoids and EPC dysfunction in diabetic patients with cardiac ischemia. Prostaglandins & Other Lipid Mediators. 2013;**100-101**:15-21

[40] Harder DR, Narayanan J, Birks EK, et al. Identification of a putative microvascular oxygen sensor. Circulation Research. 1996;**79**:54-61

[41] Katusic ZS. Vascular endothelial dysfunction: Does tetrahydrobiopterin play a role? The American Journal of Physiology. 2001;**281**:H981-H986

[42] Hink U, Li H, Mollnau H, Oelze M, Matheis E, Hartmann M, Skatchkov M, Thaiss F, Stahl RAK, Warnholtz A, Meinerz T, Griendling K, Harrison DG, Forstermann U, Munzer T. Mechanisms underlying endothelial dysfunction in diabetes mellitus. Circulation Research. 2001;**88**:E14-E22

[43] Zenere BM, Arcaro G, Saggiani F, Rossi L, Muggeo M, Lechi A. Noninvasive detection of functional alterations of the arterial wall in IDDM patients with and without microalbuminuria. Diabetes Care. 1995;**18**:975-982

[44] Gazis A, White DJ, Page SR, Cockcroft JR. Effect of oral vitamin E (alphatocopherol) supplementation on vascular endothelia lfunction in type 2 diabetes mellitus. Diabetic Medicine. 1999;**16**:304-311

[45] Bagi Z, Koller A. Lackof nitric oxide mediation of flow-dependent arteriolar dilation in type I diabetes is restored by sepiapterin. Journal of Vascular Research. 2003;**40**:47-57

[46] Drenjancevic-Peric I, Phillips SA, Falck JR, Lombard JH. Restoration of normal vascular relaxation mechanisms in cerebral arteries by chromosomal substitution in consomic SS.13BN rats. The American Journal of Physiology. 2005;**289**(1):H188-H195

[47] Misir M, Renic M, Novak S, Mihalj M, Cosic A, Vesel M, Drenjancevic I. Hyperbaric oxygenation and 20-hydroxyeicosa tetreanoic acid inhibition reduce stroke volume in female diabetic Sprague-Dawley rats. Re-Experimental Physiology. 2017;**102**(12):1596-1606

[48] Imperatore F, Cuzzocrea S, Luongo C, et al. Hyperbaric oxygen therapy prevents vascular derangement during zymosan-induced multiple-organ-failure syndrome. Intensive Care Medicine. 2004;**30**(6):1175-1181

[49] Kerkhof CJ, Bakker EN, Sipkema P. Role of cytochrome P-450 4A in oxygen sensing and NO production in rat cremaster resistance arteries. The American Journal of Physiology. 1999;**277**(4 Pt 2):H1546-H1552

[50] Phillips SA, Drenjancevic-Peric I, Frisbee JC, Lombard JH. Chronic AT(1) receptor blockade alters mechanisms mediating responses to hypoxia in rat skeletal muscle resistance arteries. American Journal of Physiology. Heart and Circulatory Physiology. 2004;**287**(2):H545-H552

[51] Alkayed NJ, Birks EK, Hudetz AG, Roman RJ, Henderson L, Harder DR. Inhibition of brain P-450 arachidonic acid epoxygenase decreases baseline cerebral blood flow. The American Journal of Physiology. 1996;**271**(4 Pt 2):H1541-H1546

[52] Liclican EL, Doumad AB, Wang J, et al. Inhibition of the adenosine2A receptor-epoxyeicosatrienoic acid pathway renders Dahl salt-resistant rats hypertensive. Hypertension. 2009;**54**:1284-1290

[53] Pozzi A, Macias-Perez I, Abair T, et al. Characterization of 5,6- and 8,9-epoxyeicosatrienoic acids (5,6- and 8,9-EET) as potent in vivo angiogenic lipids. The Journal of Biological Chemistry. 2005;**280**(29):27138-27146

[54] Xu X, Zhang XA, Wang DW. The roles of CYP450 epoxygenases and metabolites, epoxyeicosatrienoic acids, in cardiovascular and malignant diseases. Advanced Drug Delivery Reviews. 2011. Ahead of print. DOI: 10.1016/j.addr.2011.03.006

[55] Baragatti B, Ciofini E, Scebba F, et al. Cytochrome – P450 3A13 and endothelin jointly mediate ductus arteriosus constriction to oxygen in mice. American Journal of Physiology. Heart and Circulatory Physiology. 2011;**300**(3):H892-H901

[56] Lash JM, Bohlen HG. Structural and functional origins of suppressed acetylcholine vasodilation in diabetic rat intestinal arterioles. Circulation Research. 1991;**69**:1259-1268

[57] Sartoretto JL et al. Metformin treatment restores the altered microvascular reactivity in neonatal streptozotocin-induced diabetic rats increasing NOS activity,but not NOS expression. Life Sciences. 2005;**77**:2676-2689

[58] Thom SR. Hyperbaric oxygen: Its mechanisms and efficacy. Plastic and Reconstructive Surgery. 2011;**127**(Suppl 1):131S-141S

[59] Matsunami T, Sato Y, Sato T, Ariga S, Shimomura T, Yukawa M. Oxidative stress and gene expression of antioxidant enzymes in the streptozotocin-induced diabetic rats under hyperbaric oxygen exposure. International Journal of Clinical and Experimental Pathology. 2010;**3**(2):177-188

[60] Unfirer S, Drenjančević I. The mechanisms of vascular reactivity to ACh and serotonin are modulated by hyperbaric oxygen treatment in cerebral resistance arteries of diabetic rats (Pohl U, Sperandio M, editors). Journal of Vascular Research. 2011;**48**(S1):276

[61] Lombard JH, Liu Y, Fredricks KT, Bizub DM, Roman RJ, Rusch NJ. Electrical and mechanical responses of rat middle cerebral arteries to reduced PO_2 and prostacyclin. The American Journal of Physiology. 1999;**276**(2):H509-H516

[62] Feletou M, Vanhoutte PM. Chapter 4: EDHF and the physiological control of blood flow. In: EDHF: The Complete Story. Boca Raton, FL: CRC Press; 2006. pp. 133-144

[63] Unfirer S, Falck JR, Drenjancevic I. Cytochrome P450-epoxygenase metabolites play role in vasodilation of middle cerebral arteries in response to reduced pO_2 in healthy and diabetic rats that underwent hyperbaric oxygenation. In: International Union of Physiological Sciences; Birmingham, UK. July 21-26, 2013. Abstract Book. 950 p

[64] Bachi K, Puri S. Free radicals and antioxydants in health and disease. La revue de santé de la Méditerranée orientale. 1998;**4**(2):350

[65] Matsunami T, Sato Y, Hasegawa Y, Ariga S, Kashimura H, Sato T, Yukawa M. Enhancement of reactive oxygen species and induction of apoptosis in streptozotocin-induced diabetic rats under hyperbaric oxygen exposure. International Journal of Clinical and Experimental Pathology. Mar 31, 2011;**4**(3):255-266

[66] Gerber PA, Rutter GA. The role of oxidative stress and hypoxia in pancreatic beta-cell dysfunction in diabetes mellitus. Antioxidants & Redox Signaling. Apr 1, 2017;**26**(10):501-518

[67] Selim F, Wael A, Jackson KE. Diabetes-induced reactive oxygen species: Mechanism of their generation and role in renal injury. Journal of Diabetes Research. 2017;**2017**:8379327

[68] Ray PD, Huang B-W, Tsuji Y. Reactive oxygen species (ROS) homeostasis and redox regulation in cellular signaling. Cellular Signalling. May 2012;**24**(5):981-990

[69] Kirill K, Shmuel M. ROS and intracellular ion channels. Cell Calcium. Aug 2016; **60**(2):108-114

[70] Drenjancevic I, Kibel A, Kibel D, Seric V, Cosic A. Blood pressure, acid-base and blood gas status and indicators of oxidative stress in healthy male rats exposed to acute hyperbaric oxygenation. UHM Journal. 2013;**40**(4):319-328

[71] Ay H, Topal T, Uysal B, et al. Time-dependent course of hyperbaric oxygen-induced oxidative effects in rat lung and erythrocytes. Clinical and Experimental Pharmacology & Physiology. 2007;**34**:787-791

[72] Simsek K, Ay H, Topal T, et al. Long-term exposure to repetitive hyperbaric oxygen results in cumulative oxidative stress in rat lung tissue. Inhalation Toxicology. 2011;**23**:166-172

[73] Sureda A, Batle JM, Martorell M, Capó X, Tejada S, Tur JA, Pons A. Antioxidant response of chronic wounds to hyperbaric oxygen therapy. PLoS One. 2016;**11**(9):e0163371

[74] Nyoman S, Hendry I. Blood glucose and lipid profile in patients with diabetic foot ulcer that underwent hyperbaric oxygen therapy. Bali Medical Journal. 2017;**6**(2):405-408

[75] Hartge MM, Unger T, Kintscher U. The endothelium and vascular inflammation in diabetes. Diabetes & Vascular Disease Research. Jun 2007;**4**(2):84-88. PubMed PMID: 17654441

[76] Lee J, Lee S, Zhang H, Hill MA, Zhang C, Park Y. Interaction of IL-6 and TNF-alpha contributes to endothelial dysfunction in type 2 diabetic mouse hearts. PLoS One. 2017;**12**(11):e0187189. PubMed PMID: 29095915. Pubmed Central PMCID: 5667841

[77] Gustavsson C, Agardh CD, Zetterqvist AV, Nilsson J, Agardh E, Gomez MF. Vascular cellular adhesion molecule-1 (VCAM-1) expression in mice retinal vessels is affected by both hyperglycemia and hyperlipidemia. PLoS One. Sep 13, 2010;**5**(9):e12699. PubMed PMID: 20856927. Pubmed Central PMCID: 2938334

[78] Chandra SB, Mohan S, Ford BM, Huang L, Janardhanan P, Deo KS, et al. Targeted overexpression of endothelial nitric oxide synthase in endothelial cells improves cerebrovascular reactivity in Ins2Akita-type-1 diabetic mice. Journal of Cerebral Blood Flow and Metabolism: Official Journal of the International Society of Cerebral Blood Flow and Metabolism. Jun 2016;**36**(6):1135-1142. PubMed PMID: 26661212. Pubmed Central PMCID: 4908624

[79] Naguib G, Al-Mashat H, Desta T, Graves DT. Diabetes prolongs the inflammatory response to a bacterial stimulus through cytokine dysregulation. The Journal of Investigative Dermatology. Jul 2004;**123**(1):87-92. PubMed PMID: 15191547

[80] Graves DT, Naguib G, Lu H, Leone C, Hsue H, Krall E. Inflammation is more persistent in type 1 diabetic mice. Journal of Dental Research. Apr 2005;**84**(4):324-328. PubMed PMID: 15790737

[81] Khanna S, Biswas S, Shang Y, Collard E, Azad A, Kauh C, et al. Macrophage dysfunction impairs resolution of inflammation in the wounds of diabetic mice. PLoS One. Mar 4, 2010;**5**(3):e9539. PubMed PMID: 20209061. Pubmed Central PMCID: 2832020

[82] Pettersson US, Christoffersson G, Massena S, Ahl D, Jansson L, Henriksnas J, et al. Increased recruitment but impaired function of leukocytes during inflammation in mouse models of type 1 and type 2 diabetes. PLoS One. 2011;**6**(7):e22480. PubMed PMID: 21799868. Pubmed Central PMCID: 3143146

[83] Martinez N, Vallerskog T, West K, Nunes-Alves C, Lee J, Martens GW, et al. Chromatin decondensation and T cell hyperresponsiveness in diabetes-associated hyperglycemia. Journal of Immunology. Nov 1, 2014;**193**(9):4457-4468. PubMed PMID: 25246495. Pubmed Central PMCID: 4242014

[84] Wu J, Mei C, Vlassara H, Striker GE, Zheng F. Oxidative stress-induced JNK activation contributes to proinflammatory phenotype of aging diabetic mesangial cells. American Journal of Physiology Renal Physiology. Dec 2009;**297**(6):F1622-F1631. PubMed PMID: 19776174. Pubmed Central PMCID: 2801342

[85] Meng L, Park J, Cai Q, Lanting L, Reddy MA, Natarajan R. Diabetic conditions promote binding of monocytes to vascular smooth muscle cells and their subsequent differentiation. American Journal of Physiology Heart and Circulatory Physiology. Mar 2010;**298**(3):H736-H745. PubMed PMID: 20008269. Pubmed Central PMCID: 2838549

[86] Salvador B, Arranz A, Francisco S, Cordoba L, Punzon C, Llamas MA, et al. Modulation of endothelial function by Toll like receptors. Pharmacological Research. Jun 2016;**108**:46-56. PubMed PMID: 27073018

[87] Pechlivani N, Ajjan RA. Thrombosis and vascular inflammation in diabetes: Mechanisms and potential therapeutic targets. Frontiers in Cardiovascular Medicine. 2018;**5**:1. PubMed PMID: 29404341. Pubmed Central PMCID: 5780411

[88] Milovanova TN, Bhopale VM, Sorokina EM, Moore JS, Hunt TK, Hauer-Jensen M, et al. Hyperbaric oxygen stimulates vasculogenic stem cell growth and differentiation in vivo. Journal of Applied Physiology. Feb 2009;**106**(2):711-728. PubMed PMID: 19023021. Pubmed Central PMCID: 2644249

[89] Novak S, Drenjancevic I, Vukovic R, Kellermayer Z, Cosic A, Tolusic Levak M, et al. Anti-inflammatory effects of hyperbaric oxygenation during DSS-induced colitis in BALB/c mice include changes in gene expression of HIF-1alpha, proinflammatory cytokines, and antioxidative enzymes. Mediators of Inflammation. 2016;**2016**:7141430. PubMed PMID: 27656047. Pubmed Central PMCID: 5021505

[90] Kendall AC, Whatmore JL, Winyard PG, Smerdon GR, Eggleton P. Hyperbaric oxygen treatment reduces neutrophil-endothelial adhesion in chronic wound conditions through S-nitrosation. Wound Repair and Regeneration : Official Publication of the Wound Healing Society [and] The European Tissue Repair Society. Nov–Dec 2013;**21**(6):860-868. PubMed PMID: 24134224

[91] Andre-Levigne D, Modarressi A, Pignel R, Bochaton-Piallat ML, Pittet-Cuenod B. Hyperbaric oxygen therapy promotes wound repair in ischemic and hyperglycemic conditions, increasing tissue perfusion and collagen deposition. Wound Repair and Regeneration : Official Publication of the Wound Healing Society [and] The European Tissue Repair Society. Nov 2016;**24**(6):954-965. PubMed PMID: 27684570

[92] Sheikh AY, Gibson JJ, Rollins MD, Hopf HW, Hussain Z, Hunt TK. Effect of hyperoxia on vascular endothelial growth factor levels in a wound model. Archives of Surgery.. Nov 2000;**135**(11):1293-1297. PubMed PMID: 11074883

[93] Thom SR, Mendiguren I, Hardy K, Bolotin T, Fisher D, Nebolon M, et al. Inhibition of human neutrophil beta2-integrin-dependent adherence by hyperbaric O2. The American Journal of Physiology. Mar 1997;**272**(3 Pt 1):C770-C777. PubMed PMID: 9124510

[94] Benson RM, Minter LM, Osborne BA, Granowitz EV. Hyperbaric oxygen inhibits stimulus-induced proinflammatory cytokine synthesis by human blood-derived monocyte-macrophages. Clinical and Experimental Immunology. Oct 2003;**134**(1):57-62. PubMed PMID: 12974755. Pubmed Central PMCID: 1808843

[95] Kudchodkar B, Jones H, Simecka J, Dory L. Hyperbaric oxygen treatment attenuates the pro-inflammatory and immune responses in apolipoprotein E knockout mice. Clinical Immunology. Sep 2008;**128**(3):435-441. PubMed PMID: 18595776. Pubmed Central PMCID: 2562533

[96] Williams LS, Rotich J, Qi R, Fineberg N, Espay A, Bruno A, Fineberg SE, Tierney WR. Effects of admission hyperglycemia on mortality and costs in acute ischemic stroke. Neurology. 2002;**59**:67-71

[97] Kaarisalo MM, Raiha I, Sivenius J, Immonen-Raiha P, Lehtonen A, Sarti C, Mähönen M, Torppa J, Tuomilehto J, Salomaa V. Diabetes worsens the outcome of acute ischemic stroke. Diabetes Research and Clinical Practice. 2005;**69**:293-298

[98] Janghorbani M, Hu FB, Willett WC, Li TY, Manson JE, Logroscino G, Rexrode KM. Prospective study of type 1 and type 2 diabetes and risk of stroke subtypes: The nurses' health study. Diabetes Care. 2007;**30**:1730-1735

[99] Soedamah-Muthu SS, Fuller JH, Mulnier HE, Raleigh VS, Lawrenson RA, Colhoun HM. High risk of cardiovascular disease in patients with type 1 diabetes in the U.K.: A cohort study using the general practice research database. Diabetes Care. 2006;**29**:798-804

[100] Secrest AM, Prince CT, Costacou T, Miller RG, Orchard TJ. Predictors of and survival after incident stroke in type 1 diabetes. Diabetes & Vascular Disease Research. 2013;**1**:3-10

[101] Tsuruta R, Fujita M, Ono T, Koda Y, Koga Y, Yamamoto T, Nanba M, Shitara M, Kasaoka S, Maruyama I, et al. Hyperglycemia enhances excessive superoxide anion radical generation, oxidative stress, early inflammation, and endothelial injury in forebrain ischemia/reperfusion rats. Brain Research. 2010;**1309**:155-163

[102] Powers WJ, Rabinstein AA, Ackerson T, Adeoye OM, Bambakidis NC, Becker K, biller J, Brown M, Demaerschalk BM, Hoh B, Jauch EC, Kidwell CS, Leslie-Mazwi TM, Ovbiagele B, Scott PA, Sheth KN, Southerland AM, Summers DV, Tirschwell DL; American Heart Association Stroke Council. Guidelines for the Early Management of Patients with Acute Ischemic Stroke: A Guideline for Healthcare Professionals from the American Heart Association/American Stroke Association. Stroke 2018;**49**:46-110

[103] Xu RS. Pathogenesis of diabetic cerebral vascular disease complication. World Journal of Diabetes. 2015;**6**(1):54-66

[104] Michalski D, Hartig W, Schneider D, Hobohm C. Use of normobaric and hyperbaric oxygen in acute focal cerebral ischemia-a preclinical and clinical review. Acta Neurologica Scandinavica. 2011;**123**:85-97

[105] Sunami K, Takeda Y, Hashimoto M, et al. Hyperbaric oxygen reduces infarct volume in rats by increasing oxygen supply to the ischemic periphery. Critical Care Medicine. 2000;**28**:2831-2836

[106] Liu S, Liu W, Ding W, et al. Electron paramagnetic resonance-guided normobarichyperoxia treatment protects the brain by maintaining penumbral oxygenation in a rat model of transient focal cerebral ischemia. Journal of Cerebral Blood Flow and Metabolism. 2006;**26**:1274-1284

[107] Singhal AB. A review of oxygen therapy in ischemic stroke. Neurological Research. 2007;**29**:173-183

[108] Lou M, Eschenfelder CC, Herdegen T, Brecht S, Deuschl G. Therapeutic window for use of hyperbaric oxygenation in focal transient ischemia in rats. Stroke. 2004;**35**:578-583

[109] Singhal AB, Lo EH, Dalkara T, et al. Advances in stroke neuroprotection: Hyperoxia and beyond. Neuroimaging Clinics of North America. 2005;**15**:697-720

[110] Zhai WW, Sun L, Yu ZQ, Chen G. Hyperbaric oxygen therapy in experimental and clinical stroke. Medical Gas Research. 2016;**6**:111-118

[111] Mišir M, Renić M, Mihalj M, Novak S, Drenjančević I. Is shorter transient middle cerebral artery occlusion (t-MCAO) duration better in stroke experiments on diabetic female Sprague Dawely rats? Brain Injury. 2016;**30**:1390-1396

[112] Nagasawa H, Kogure K. Correlation between cerebral blood flow and histologic changes in a new rat model of middle cerebral artery occlusion. Stroke. 1989;**20**:1037-1043

[113] Xu Y, Ji R, Wei R, et al. The efficacy of hyperbaric oxygen therapy on middle cerebral artery occlusion in animal studies: A meta-analysis (Pignataro G, editor.) PLoS One. 2016;**11**:e0148324

[114] Bennett MH, Wasiak J, Schnabel A, et al. Hyperbaric oxygen therapy for acute ischaemic stroke. Cochrane Database of Systematic Reviews. 2005;**3**:CD004954

Chapter 7

Toxic Effects of Hyperbaric Conditions

Ali Erdal Gunes

Additional information is available at the end of the chapter

http://dx.doi.org/10.5772/intechopen.78392

Abstract

Hyperbaric oxygen therapy is highly safe in treatments based on internationally accepted treatment tables. However, in some long-term treatments, the internal adjuvant and the patient are exposed to some toxic effects. In the presence of compressed air environment, nitrogen can lead to drunkenness. Another cause of poisoning is oxygen. Oxygen shows toxic effects when inhaled in the high-pressure environment for long periods or above partial pressures on 3 ATA. The excess oxygen has a toxic effect on the lung and central nervous system (CNS). Oxygen poisoning can be seen in long-term oxygen therapy in intensive care, in closed or semi-closed circuit diving, in saturation dives, on decompressions on the surface, in recompression and hyperbaric oxygen therapy. The first goal during convulsion is to prevent trauma prevent the patient from biting his tongue during the seizure. However, in nitrogen narcosis, the first intervention should be to prevent the diver from diving deeper to reduce the effect of anesthesia. The lifeguard must prevent the unconscious movements of the diver, such as removing the regulator from his mouth and holding his breath. He must think that the dive is like a dream.

Keywords: hyperbaric oxygenation, toxic actions, neurotoxicity syndromes, acute lung injury

1. Introduction

Inert gases are shown to have an effect in the body without entering metabolic and chemical activities [1]. The inert gas, which is nitrogen, encountered with problems in sports equipped divers. For this reason, what is known as inert gas narcosis in diving medicine can be called direct nitrogen narcosis in this chapter [2].

Nitrogen narcosis, depth poisoning, depth drunkenness, nitrogen narcosis is also known by other names [1]. The nitrogen that the two nitrogen molecules bind with three bonds between them constitutes 79% of the air we breathe [3]. The increase of the nitrogen pressure negatively affects the central nervous system (CNS). It is usually seen at depths of more than 30 m [4]. Nitrogen narcosis is characterized by decreased intellectual function and decreased neuromuscular transmission performance, a tendency to laugh, decreased attention and decision-making, emotional state, and impaired behavior. Nitrogen narcosis does not cause permanent damage to the body, but mental and motor deterioration can lead to serious problems in the underwater [2]. These effects increase as the partial pressure of nitrogen increases, but it is not related to the time remaining at the same depth [5]. These changes have been seen for centuries as they are known when diving with compressed air due to nitrogen pressure. Other inert gases with similar effects have been described (neon, argon, krypton, xenon, and hydrogen) [1].

In diving with compressed air, nitrogen narcosis is the most important factor limiting depth. When it is necessary to work deeper than 40–50 m, it is necessary to get help from gas with less narcotic effect such as helium. Nitrogen narcosis is responsible for most of the dive accidents and dive-related deaths.

The cause of acute toxicity of hyperbaric oxygen therapy is related to oxygen partial pressure [6]. Although oxygen is a necessary gas to survive, oxygen can show toxic effects at high partial pressures and long-term exposures. Oxygen poisoning can be seen in long-term oxygen therapy in intensive care, in closed or semi-closed circuit diving, in saturation dives, on decompressions on the surface, in recompression and hyperbaric oxygen therapy [7].

Oxygen intoxication is caused by reactions between free oxygen radicals and cell components [8]. Gamma amino butyric acid (GABA) has frequently been studied in studies conducted in this regard [9]. Excess oxygen causes the generation of uncontrolled stimuli in the central nervous system by reducing GABA outflows [8]. It is thought that seizures developing in 3 ATA and above hyperbaric oxygen therapy are related to this [10].

2. History

The poisoning caused by air inhalation in a high-pressure environment was first described by Junod in 1835 [2]. In 1861, Green made a dive with divers with 48 m of compressed air, observing that the divers developed to sleep, their decision-making powers were impaired, and they saw hallucinations. Paul Bert stated that divers were poisoned at high depths in 1878. In 1903, Hill and McLeod described the intellectual functions of tunnel workers as inadequate at 5.5 ATA pressure. In 1930, Damant reported that memory problems had developed in 10 ATA. In 1932, Hill and Phillips thought these effects could be claustrophobic or psychological. According to a report by the British Navy in 1933, the section entitled "Loss of semi-consciousness" states that divers who have dived at 60–106 m have received hand signals sent to them, but no one remembers it when it comes to the surface [1].

In 1935, Behnke and his colleagues described the currently accepted theory of nitrogen narcosis. Narcosis is caused by an increase in partial pressure of nitrogen, which is an inert gas. The

http://dx.doi.org/10.5772/intechopen.78392

enthusiasm (euphoria) developed at the 30-m compressed air dive; accompany slowing of the mental capacity and deterioration of the nerve-muscle communication. Attention was paid to the fact that this effect was further enhanced by the depth of the dive. At diving, drowsiness occurs at 90 m and loss of consciousness occurs at 90–140 m. Behnke and Yarbrough reported that this effect could be reduced by replacing nitrogen to helium in the dive inhalation gas [1].

According to the Deep Dive Committee Report in 1933, this was also related to the accumulation of carbon dioxide during the dive. In 1941, Case and Haldane showed that, when carbon dioxide was mixed in the diving air, the mental symptoms became more intense. However, In some studies clearly denied the carbon dioxide theory. They showed evidence of narcotic symptoms despite normal levels of carbon dioxide in the alveolar air. In subsequent years of studies has been found that direct anesthesia is responsible for the nitrogen between the air and dive with helium/oxygen [2].

3. Etiology

It is thought that the mechanism of nitrogen narcosis is the same as general anesthesia with volatile gases. All inert gases that produce anesthetic effects behave in the same way. These gases are composed of simple molecules with no structural properties and do not show chemical changes in the body [3].

Many researchers have attempted to understand the physical behavior of these gases and have found a close relationship with the oil dissolution feature. According to the Meyer-Overton hypothesis, there is a parallel between the dissolution of anesthetics in oil and potency of the narcotic effect. It stated that when the gases pass through cell oils at a certain molar concentration, they will show an effect of narcosis. In this case, the inert gas molecule affects the cell membrane function in the brain. However, there are some discrepancies in terms of the physical properties of the inert gases and their narcotics abilities (**Table 1**). For example, argon is two times more narcotic than nitrogen. However, their fat/water solubility ratios are similar. However, despite all these incompatibilities, narcotic behavior is parallel to physical characteristics in general [5].

According to Henry's Law, as soon as the partial pressure of nitrogen increases, it begins to dissolve more in the body and in the plasma. Nitrogen cannot be used by the body like oxygen. When we breathe compressed air during diving, many molecules enter our bodies and quickly dissolve in our bodies due to the height of the environmental pressure. When we dive 15 m sea water, the nitrogen partial pressure will double up. With the increase in depth, the narcosis signs will begin to appear. As is known, anesthetic symptoms occur when diving is 15 m or more, and we briefly explain it with the Martini Act (**Figure 1**) [4].

The dissolution hypothesis in oil has been tried to be understood by the concept of critical volume. Here, in order to develop the effect of narcosis, the inert gas must affect on the fat part of cell membrane to swell. In human studies, it has been confirmed that gas has a positive correlation with oil solubility by developing slightly to moderate narcosis.

Gases	Molecular weight	Volume	Solubility in oil at 37°C	Separation coefficient (oil:water)	narcotic effect
Helium	4	2.370	0.015	1.70	0.23
Neon	20	1.709	0.019	2.07	0.28
Hydrogen	2	2.661	0.040	3.10	0.55
Nitrogen	28	3.913	0.067	5.25	1.00
Argon	40	3.218	0.140	5.32	2.33
Krypton	83.7	3.978	0.430	9.60	7.14
Xenon	131.3	3.105	1.700	20.00	25.64

Table 1. Narcotic effects and physical properties of some gases.

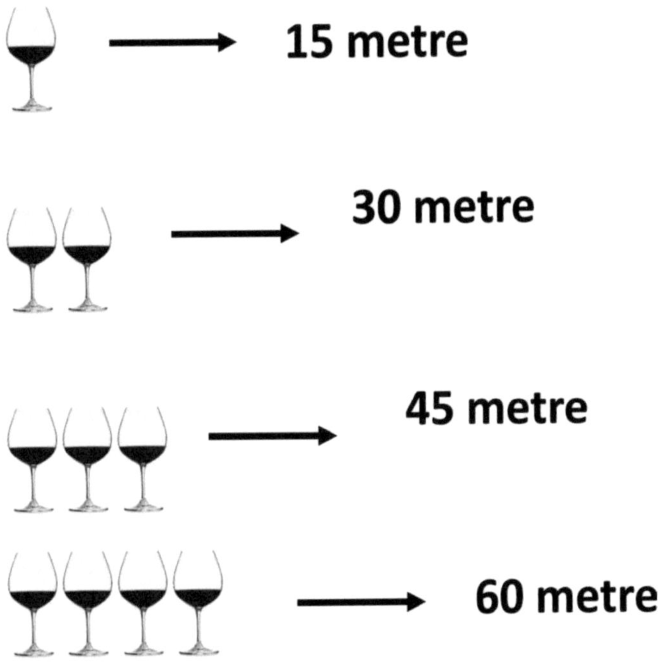

Figure 1. Martini Yasası.

In general, although these physical theories refer to the fatty part of the cell membrane, it has been shown that this narcotic effect is due to specific receptors and influences synaptic transmission. Some studies have shown that cell membranes are resistant to narcotics and cell membrane proteins and lipoproteins are responsible for this.

http://dx.doi.org/10.5772/intechopen.78392

Many studies have focused on the cause of stimulation in the central nervous system. Stimulant-inhibitory synapses, molecules, and receptors are the basis of this effect. Among them, gamma-amyno butiric acid (GABA) is the most important inhibitory molecule. GABA is an important inhibitory neurotransmitter which made from glutamine after a series of reactions in the central nervous system (**Figure 2**). GABA receptors have been shown to be responsible for the formation of nitrogen narcosis [8].

The most important of the stimulating molecules is dopamine. Nitrogen accumulation increases the levels of dopamine, causing cortex and thalamus stimulation, which are brain regions (**Figure 3**). Nitrogen accumulation causes a reversal of uptake and an increase in dopaminergic levels. This situation leads to stimulation in the thalamus and striatum, which is the inhibitor center. This explains some neuromuscular disorders belonging to nitrogen narcosis [9].

In order to explain the acute toxic effects of hyperbaric oxygen therapy, it is necessary to focus on enzyme metabolism. High pO_2 values disrupt the function of enzymes, especially those containing sulfurized sulfhydryl groups. This effect of free oxygen radicals is widely accepted [7].

For example, the antioxidant defense system in the body can resist life to the oxygen pressure normally found in atmospheric air, or even slightly more. This value is 0.4–0.5 atmospheres (1 ATA at sea level, oxygen is approximately one-fifth in the air). Now, let's take a 30-m dive with air. In this case, total pressure will be 4 ATA, and if the oxygen forming partial pressure of air is pO_2 = 0.8 ATA, this value exceeds the antioxidant defense system of the body. The body is damaged acutely by oxygen at a depth of 30 m for a long time.

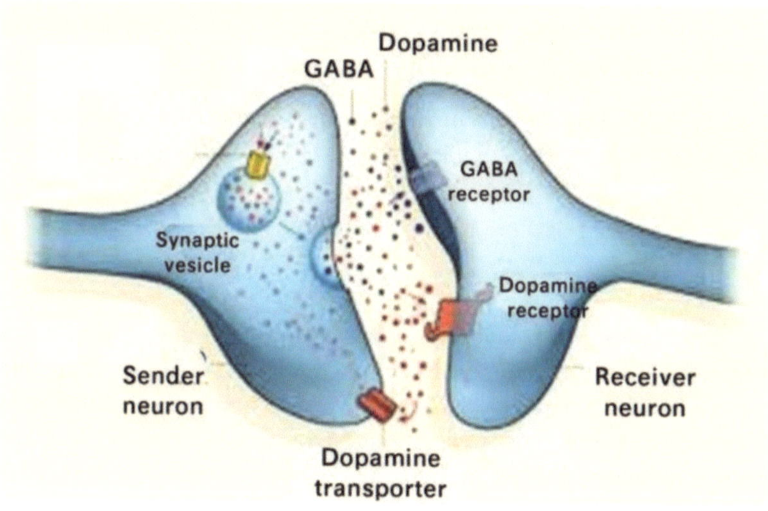

Figure 2. GABA and dopamine metabolism.

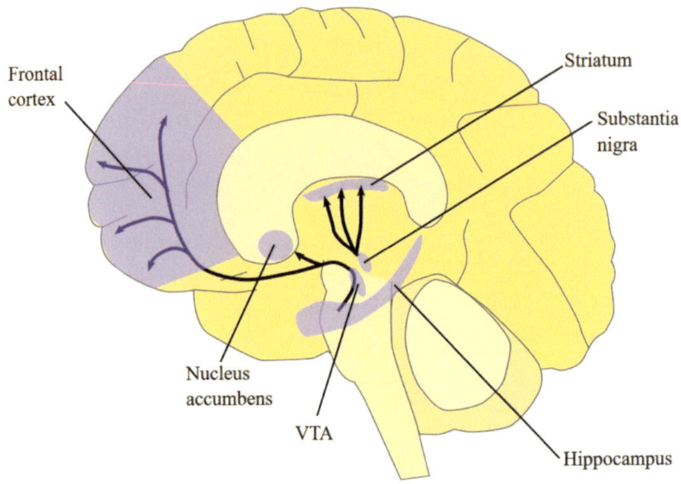

Figure 3. Dopamine-induced thalamus and cortex.

4. Theories

- *Myer-Overton:* when inert gas is dissolved in the nervous system, the inert gas has an inhibitory effect on the nervous system.

- *Quastel-Metabolic:* at high pressure, inert gas disrupts cell metabolism. These sensitive cells are mostly found in the brain. The cells, which are consciousness formation, are the first to be affected.

- *Clathrate:* under pressure nitrogen creates clathrate with protein and water. This formation disrupts neural transmission.

- *Iceberg:* when nitrogen gas dissolves in water, it creates molecules called icebergs. The iceberg also prevents the transmission of the nervous system like the same clathrate [4].

5. Pathophysiology

There are many variables that affect the susceptibility of the person to nitrogen narcosis. Diving health, deep diving experience, working conditions, environmental conditions are some of these. As the depth increases, the diver starts sign of the suppressing. Thinking problems, deterioration of time perception, deterioration of decision-making, memory problems, motor and mental functions, and the prolongation of reaction time are some of these [5].

When the diver starts to exit, the symptoms disappear quickly; sometimes, it does not remember what you are doing underwater during nitrogen narcosis.

There is no direct pathological change to acutely CNS oxygen poisoning in humans. In animal experiments, tissue death was demonstrated in the nervous system. Serious exposures can cause damage to the brain and spinal cord in the spinal cord. Even a 30-min dive with 4 ATA pure oxygen (30 m) can cause structural changes in the gray matter in the spine of front horn [7].

6. Clinical signs and symptoms

The mechanism of CNS oxygen poisoning is not fully known. Oxygen is believed to have evolved by the increase of pO_2 and the free oxygen derivatives affecting the CNS metabolism. As a rule, poisoning is seen when exposed to pO_2 pressure on 2 ATA and above [6].

Oxygen poisoning occurs more rapidly as the pO_2 pressure increases. According to Clark and Lambertsen's work; pO_2 1.7 ATA for 7 h, 1.8 ATA for 3 h, 2 ATA for 50 min and 3 ATA for 30 min showed signs of MSS poisoning [7].

Signs and findings are described in a wide range of fans. Nausea, vomiting, dizziness, ringing in the ears, incoordination, tunnel vision, irritability, pallor, sweating, heart rate slowing (bradycardia), lips, and hands twitching, eyes widening of the baby, hiccups, to remember the recent past, hallucination, confusion (confusion) are chief of the signs and findings. However, the most dramatic of these is the seizure, namely the convulsion. It is typical that consciousness is closed during convulsion [7].

The most common finding is a face twenty in the oxygen pressure on 2 ATA. The sign of paleness in the face is due to hyperoxia-induced vasoconstriction. Similarly, the loss of sensation in the fingers is the result of vasoconstriction [9].

Even though the depth is the same, being in the water reduces the resistance to oxygen poisoning considerably compared to being in dry air in the pressure chamber. Water and diving stress increase the susceptibility to oxygen poisoning. Also underwater, the signs mentioned above cannot be noticed, but the divers are noticed that they are poisoned when they have convulsions. Convulsions underwater are dangerous because they can lead to suffocation or barotrauma. Therefore, many authorities have determined the maximum depth of pure oxygen diving underwater to be 10 m. Other causes that reduce the threshold value of CNS poisoning are exercise, hypothermia, increased calm carbon dioxide levels [10].

Facial twitch usually results in convulsions. During convulsion, all body stimuli develop and the tonic phase called full contraction begins. During this time, breathing is interrupted. The tonic phase usually lasts 30 s and is accompanied by loss of consciousness. This period approximately takes 1 min, followed by the head, neck, trunk, and legs in large contraction followed by clonic phase. After the clonic phase, the contractures decrease and the respiration starts with hyperventilation, and after a while consciousness comes back. The diver does not remember any part of the event. The concentration of carbon dioxide has increased because of being held breath during the convulsion. However, contrary to normal epilepsy patients, there is no reduction in oxygen reaching the CNS during respiration, as oxygen breathes at high pressure before the diver seizure [11].

When toxic effects of oxygen occur, it is necessary to reduce the partial pressure of oxygen inhaled immediately. In the pressure chamber, it is necessary to remove the oxygen mask or reduce the pressure. Diving depth must be reduced during diving. The diver must be brought to the surface safely. Reducing the pressure in the pressure chamber or rising in the dive is accompanied by lung barotrauma risk because it is kept breath during the seizure. After first aid, barotrauma should be controlled by drawing a chest radiograph [8].

Although the sensitivity of nitrogen narcosis is quite different from person to person, all the divers who dive at depths of 60–70 m demonstrate clinical signs of nitrogen narcosis. Firstly, high cognitive functions are affected. The main symptoms of these are judgments, decision-making, close memory, learning, concentration, and attention. The diver may feel very good and can over-confidence himself as a light alcohol drinker. Along with increased nitrogen partial pressure at higher pressures, diminished hand strength and progressive deterioration of mental performance, intellectual fixation, hallucinations, and finally lethargy/blunting and coma. Some divers may experience a disorder in the form of tunnel vision, but they cannot be aware of the danger because of the perception disorder [1].

Tension, cold, tiredness, soothing medicines, alcohol and medications that affect the central nervous system may cause exacerbated narcosis. The effects of nitrogen narcosis are likened to the intake of alcohol. Alcohol and nitrogen narcosis symptoms are often associated, especially as enthusiasm and motor coordination develop. Even with a somewhat sarcastic approach, the nitrogen narcosis is assessed with a criterion called the Martini law. According to this law, every 50 feet of depth leads to equivalent effects on a glass of martin. Enthusiasm, joy, laughter at 10–30 m; increased self-confidence, fixed idea at 30–50 m; loquaciousness, dizziness, hysterical seizures at 50–70 m; delayed response to stimuli, loss of concentration, mood swings at 70–90 m; hallucinations, and loss of consciousness develop over 90 m [3].

The nitrogen narcosis effect is affected within a few minutes when you descend into depth and is not related to the dive time. Initially, fast diving increases the anesthetic effect, but this effect is rapidly returned when ascending to surface [3].

Other causes that increase the degree of nitrogen narcosis need to be considered. Alcohol, fatigue, tension, cold, oxygen, and carbon dioxide changes increase the effect of narcosis, limiting the diver's ability in underwater. Experimental studies have shown that alcohol and underwater exercises increase the effect of narcosis. Increased carbon dioxide and nitrogen pressurized diver have been shown to reduce performance. In certain periods and long dives, divers can develop some adaptations against to the narcotic effect of nitrogen [4].

Despite the fact that it is not a realistic and appropriate guide for the formation of nitrogen narcosis, scientific studies are carrying out. It is useful to monitor the performance of the diver in simple tasks, tests that can be reached to narcotic sensitive individuals, the use of low narcotic gas mixtures during diving and reduction of other factors affecting narcosis in depth, achieve a safe dive operation without encountering this effect. Since these tests are not used in the selection of the sportive diver or mixed gas is not used in sportive diving, the depth of the dive is reduced or terminated when anesthesia develops. It is also necessary to

http://dx.doi.org/10.5772/intechopen.78392

pay attention to the other factors, which increase the influence of nitrogen narcosis mentioned in the previous paragraph. The effects of nitrogen narcosis are roughly measured by two methods. First of these, the behavioral approach measures the fulfillment of the assigned task, which measures arithmetic, memory, and handicraft. The other is a measure of some neurophysiological parameters [5].

(A) Behavioral approach

The behavioral approach is examined in three main categories: cognitive ability, reaction time, and skill. Cognitive competence is the most frequently affected by nitrogen narcosis, but skill competence is least affected.

In this study, conducted on open water divers, anxiety, and a decrease in the success of the task were observed. The anxiety status was determined by measuring plasma cortisol and urine noradrenaline. The intellectual function, arithmetic, and memory capacity of open dives were found lower than the coastal diving in open sea diving. The cause of this decline is depending on stress of the open sea diving.

The effect of nitrogen narcosis on behavior has been studied by psychologists. They defined this as a slow process model. In this model, they saw slowed activation with anesthesia, increased reactivation duration. The least affected hand is skill because less cognitive function is needed for skill.

(B) Neurophysiological changes

Neurophysiological tests are needed to evaluate some subjective values, to achieve low performance and to provide objective evidence. These are the information that is obtained by drawing the electroencephalogram of the brain after diving with compressed air in the cabin. First, findings of high stimulation in the cortex of the brain have been reached. This situation includes voltage increases in the basal rhythm of the brain.

The measurement of the functions of the central nervous system can be done by examining the cortical potentials, evoked from the exposed inert gases in the brain. The low response to stimulus is an experimental measure of the effect of nitrogen narcosis.

7. Treatment

When acute poisoning statements are made during treatment in the pressure chamber, the patient should be given air to breathe deeply. If necessary, the treatment table can be changed by the underwater physician. In case of unconsciousness, stomach contents should be prevented from escaping to the lungs (aspiration).

The first goal during convulsion is to prevent trauma [7]. The tongue should prevent the patient from biting the tongue during the seizure. It should be known that naturally depends on the dive, the lack of oxygen (hypoxia) does not occur. It is necessary to wait until the tonic phase of the convulsion is finished. Otherwise, the diver may be exposed to lung barotrauma.

If oxygen poisoning develops in the pressure chamber treatment;

- Stop diving, remove the mask.
- If convulsion develops, it will prevent damage to itself and its surroundings.
- Tongue bite is blocked by attendance.
- Enables hyperventilation with air in the pressure chamber.
- The sedative drug can be started with the recommendation of the underwater physician.
- If symptoms have disappeared after interruption of treatment within 15 minutes, it will be resumed from the same point of treatment.
- If necessary proceed to non-deeper treatment tables.

The first intervention should be to prevent the diver from deeper to reduce the effect of anesthesia. The lifeguard must prevent the unconscious movements of the diver, such as removing the regulator from his mouth and holding his breath. He must think that the dive is like a dream, and he should try to go to ascend from the depth.

The diver must be closely followed when he comes out of the water. There is no treatment to be done when the anesthetic effect is passed. During close follow-up, hypoxic findings, drowning, sudden outbreaks, etc. should be considered and examined for secondary problems. The underwater physician should be consulted if such cases are found to be present.

8. Prevention

When medications that prevent convulsions are used before the dive, the convulsion is under control, but cell damage is still present. This causes the diver to reach uncontrolled depths and be exposed to more toxic effects. The only safe approach is to make diving plans at depth limits. This limit depends on the partial pressure of the oxygen, the duration of the dive and environmental factors.

Underwater physicians test the candidates who are susceptible to CNS oxygen poisoning. The oxygen tolerance test can be done by oxygen breathing in the hyperbaric oxygen therapy device at 2.8 ATM for 30 min. Although this test is susceptible to positive ones, there is no clinical validity of the "oxygen tolerance test." Tolerance can vary from person to person or from day to day in the same person [9].

In the simplest case, it is necessary to avoid high partial pressures of inert gases during diving. It is important to be aware of the circumstances of air diving and know that performance and decision-making authority will be affected at depths of over 40 m. In professional diving, it is necessary to use less narcotic gases such as helium to increase the depth of safe diving. It is known that the adaptation of the dive with the daily dives against nitrogen narcosis. Some studies have shown that although some personal adaptations can occur, reaction times do not benefit from repeated dives.

To prevent nitrogen narcosis, some mixed gases are used in professional dives. Diving is planned here by creating a mixture of oxygen with nitrogen, helium or helium/nitrogen. The aim here is to reduce the narcotic effect by reducing the partial pressure of the nitrogen. However, it is necessary to pay careful attention to oxygen poisoning since oxygen increases partial pressure in such diving. As helium increases heat transfer, divers must be careful against the hypothermic effect. Due to such effects, only professional divers are allowed to mix gas dives.

Amphetamines reduce the narcotic effect that causes the prolongation of the reaction period, so they are not used in diving. The diver should be aware of the risks in the underwater environment. Also, increase narcotic efficacy, drugs that suppress the central nervous system, such as alcohol and antihistamines. These drugs create a synergistic effect with nitrogen, accelerating the reduction of performance and decision-making.

9. Return to diving

When the symptoms disappear, and the diver feels ready, the dive may return. It should be noted here that nitrogen is a secondary health problem that will develop in a diver who is forced to exit during narcosis. If necessary, the diver should be re-examined [2].

In diving accidents, the treatment of hypoxic injuries is more important than oxygen poisoning. Therefore, priority should be given to the treatment of diving accidents. In the treatment of decompression, air or gas mixtures can be used in the pressure chamber to reduce the most toxic damage. Vitamin A, C, E, selenium, and so on to reduce oxygen poisoning. Antioxidant products can be used in hyperbaric oxygen therapy or before diving [7].

Author details

Ali Erdal Gunes

Address all correspondence to: aerdalg@gmail.com

Department of Underwater and Hyperbaric Clinical Medicine, Faculty of Medicine, Harran University, Sanliurfa, Turkey

References

[1] Lowry C. Inert gas narcosis. In: Edmonds C, Lowry C, Pennefather J, Walker R, editors. Diving and Subaquatic Medicine. 4th ed. London: Arnold Publ; 2002. pp. 183-193

[2] Strauss MB, Aksenov IM. The inert gas load. In: Strauss MB, Aksenov IM, editors. Diving Sicence. 1st ed. USA: Human Kinetics; 2004. pp. 51-80

[3] Bennett PB, Rostain JC. Inert gas narcosis. In: Bennett PB, Cronje FC, Campbell ES, editors. Assessment of Diving Medical Fitness for Scuba Divers and Instructors. 1st ed. Canada: Best Publishing; 2006. pp. 300-322

[4] Edmonds CE. Nitrogen narcosis. In: Edmonds CE, McKenzie B, Thomas R, Pennefather J, editors. Diving Medicine For Scuba Divers. 6th ed. Australia: Carl Edmonds; 2015. (Chapter 18)

[5] Bosco G, Rizzato A, Moon RE, Camporesi EM. Environmental physiology and diving medicine. Frontiers in Psychology. 2018;**9**:72

[6] Lowry C. Oxygen toxicity. In: Edmonds C, Lowry C, Pennefather J, Walker R, editors. Diving and Subaquatic Medicine. 4th ed. London: Arnold Publ; 2002. pp. 207-222

[7] Çimşit M. Hiperbarik Tıp, Teori ve Uygulama. Ankara: Eflatun Yayınevi; 2009. pp. 71-86

[8] Strauss MB, Aksenov IM. Bottom problems. In: Strauss MB, Aksenov IM, editors. Diving Sicence. 1st ed. USA: Human Kinetics; 2004. p. 270

[9] Bennett PB, Cronje FC, Campbell ES. Gases and decompression. In: Bennett PB, Cronje FC, Campbell ES, editors. Assesment of Diving Medical Fitness for Scuba Divers and Instructors. 1st ed. Canada: Best Publishing; 2006. pp. 14-16

[10] Edmonds CE. Oxygen toxicity. In: Edmonds CE, McKenzie B, Thomas R, Pennefather J, editors. Diving Medicine For Scuba Divers. 6th ed. Australia: Carl Edmonds; 2015. (Chapter 21)

[11] van Ooij PA, Sterk PJ, van Hulst RA. Oxygen, the lung and the diver: Friends and foes? European Respiratory Review. 2016;**25**(142):496-505